CENTR
828 "I" STREET
SACRAMENTO, CA 95814

FAT CHAT
with TAMARA

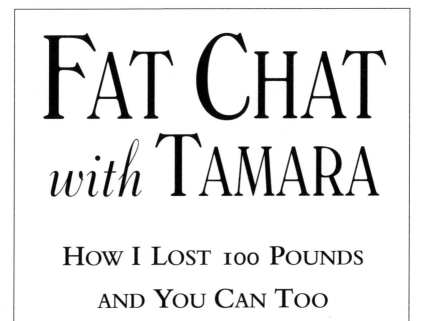

FAT CHAT
with TAMARA

HOW I LOST 100 POUNDS
AND YOU CAN TOO

TAMARA HILL
with MARYANN BRINLEY

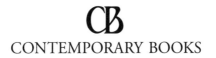

CONTEMPORARY BOOKS

Library of Congress Cataloging-in-Publication Data

Hill, Tamara.
    Fat chat with Tamara : how I lost 100 pounds and you can too / Tamara Hill
with Maryann Brinley.
        p.   cm.
    ISBN 0-8092-2605-7
    1. Weight loss.   2. Physical fitness.   I. Brinley, Maryann Bucknum.
    II. Title
    RM222.2.H476   2000
    613.7—dc21   99-54853
                                                                          CIP

Cover design by Kim Bartko
Cover photograph by Deborah Whitlaw
Interior design by Scott Rattray

Published by Contemporary Books
A division of NTC/Contemporary Publishing Group, Inc.
4255 West Touhy Avenue, Lincolnwood (Chicago), Illinois 60712-1975 U.S.A.
Printed in the United States of America
International Standard Book Number: 0-8092-2605-7
00 01 02 03 04 05 MV 15 14 13 12 11 10 9 8 7 6 5 4 3 2 1

Contents

Introduction   vii

Acknowledgments   xi

To Lose 100 Pounds . . .

1. "I Found the Truth About the Diet Industry's
   Losing Game"   1

2. "I Became Accountable to Me and Only Me"   15

3. "I Simply Started Moving"   27

4. "I Focused on My Positive Points"   41

5. "I Learned There Is Nothing Evil About Food"   53

6. "I Discovered That Small Changes Are
   Always Better than None"   67

7. "I Began to Love How My Body Moved"   79

8. "I Knew for Sure That the Miracle Was
   in My Mind"   93

9. "Now It's Your Turn"
   To Lose 100 Pounds . . .   109

Resources   143

Additional Reading   145

Introduction

Don't skip this introduction. You need fair warning as well as a literary road map to handle the journey you are about to begin. Otherwise, you might get lost, and I certainly don't want to lose any readers on this trip.

When I was half the distance to completing a manuscript about Tamara Hill's Fat Chat program based in Augusta, Georgia, I tossed about 30,000 words into the trash. No kidding. What I had written was not really all that horrible; no, what made me want to throw those words away was the fact that they were so predictable and not nearly inspiring enough.

If you are like millions of other readers, you may already know a lot about what you need to do to lose weight. What's missing is the motivation. Almost every book about weight loss offers a program that will make you feel guilty unless you follow it religiously. Eventually, the programs lead to feelings of failure. That was where I was heading with that first incomplete draft of a book: an intense focus on the Fat Chat with Tamara program that might have led you to guilt and just another loss in that war with your body. Yet, I couldn't shake the fact that when I was in Tamara Hill's presence, guilt and failure were nowhere to be seen.

I needed a format that would draw you into her life and give you unpredictable glimpses of what it might be like to be there physically in her sessions. I also wanted you to spend some personal, quality time walking in her shoes . . . as she lost 100 pounds. Her journey from obesity to fitness was not the result of a structured week-by-week, point-by-point, or one-two-three approach to lifestyle changes. You can't copy every little step she made or eat exactly as she ate and expect to lose 100 pounds. However, when I examined the evidence behind her success, I discovered that there were simple secrets that she had stumbled upon and on which her program is based. These eight easy notions are so basic that they may make you want to laugh out loud. "Hah," you snort! But don't be too cynical. Take it from me: they work.

In each of eight sections, you will meet The Person. Of course, this person is Tamara Hill, the founder of Fat Chat and the individual who may become the catalyst to changing your life. I've tried to paint her personality for you by using biographical bits, anecdotes, snippets of conversations, and feedback from Fat Chat participants and admirers. Tamara and I also thought that it might be fun for you to be able to place yourself right there with us, through descriptions of the scenes in which our chat sessions occurred. That's why you'll see datelines.

You'll also encounter The Program, a subhead that will alert you to the fact that Tamara is about to lead you in a new way of thinking about yourself, exercising, or eating. She's teaching, coaching, or cheerleading in these sections but not always in the hospital, the gym, or the classroom. Once, I caught her in a church, and sometimes lessons arrive via telephone conversations, at a kitchen table, or over the radio.

The third main element under each of the eight simple secrets is Tamara's Journey . . . in Her Own Words, which tells the story of her weight loss and journey to wellness. Throughout the book, we've also included brief quotes, excerpts, and epigrams to keep your inspiration level as high as possible and to add other voices of reason to the discussion.

The ninth chapter, "Now It's Your Turn . . . ," will expose you to typical sixteen-week sessions of Fat Chat with Tamara. Her program originated in Augusta and is currently offered at a local hospital, a gym, and a fitness studio, but the possible variations on this sixteen-week format are endless. As she says often, "I don't care if you have sixteen weeks, sixteen days, or sixteen minutes. That's not important." Because most people can't hop onto a plane and head for Augusta, we thought you might want to see the kinds of ingredients others are using to create their very own individualized wellness plans.

Not every single aerobic exercise is included in the book, because it's up to you to find the ones you like to do in your own circle of everyday life. Likewise, not every pointer about eating healthily is included, because Tamara expects you to be able to go out there and find what works best for your own body. In fact, Fat Chat with Tamara is designed to help you redesign your own life. As Tamara says often, "If I can change my life, so can you too. You can rewrite your own story."

MARYANN BUCKNUM BRINLEY

Acknowledgments

THIS BOOK IS dedicated to two very important men in my life: my father, also known to many as Poppa, and my oldest brother, Ed.

Seven years ago, Poppa brought me to the end of the tunnel. He helped me turn on the light. He taught me that nothing is more important than my health. He helped me to learn to love myself through the unconditional love he showed me. Even when he was stricken with cancer a second time, Poppa was still there for me. His undying love helped me emotionally through two military court martials with my ex-husband. Poppa traveled from Minnesota in the fall of 1997 and stayed with my children and me until he died in June of 1998. Without the continued emotional, physical, spiritual, and financial help of Poppa, there would be no Fat Chat with Tamara. He believed in me and the Fat Chat mission.

Since Poppa's death, my brother Ed, who resides in Buffalo, Minnesota, has taken up where Poppa left off. Ed has truly become my guardian angel here on earth. Despite severe heart problems, he continues to be here for me, and Fat Chat, emotionally, spiritually, and financially. Brother, thank you so much for your continued love and support.

A special thank-you also goes to my sister Sharon, of Clovis, California, for her continued love and prayers for the Fat Chat mission.

TAMARA K. HILL

To Bob, Zach, Maggie, all my supporters in the Bucknum and Brinley clans, my agent, Agnes Birnbaum of Bleecker Street Associates, Gay Norton Edelman of *McCall's*, my Contemporary Books editor Kara Leverte, and Sue Gleason for all of our "tennis lessons" . . . Whew!

MARYANN BUCKNUM BRINLEY

FAT CHAT
with TAMARA

To Lose 100 Pounds . . .

"I Found the Truth About the Diet Industry's Losing Game"

The Person

A wise man has a simple wisdom
Which other men seek.
Without taking credit
Is accredited.
Laying no claim
Is acclaimed.

TAOIST PROVERB

My Third-Floor Office in Upper Montclair, New Jersey:

I AVOIDED MAKING the phone call for weeks. A book about weight loss! A book about fitness! A book about healthy eating! A book about learning to love your body! Yeah, sure. No way. There are thousands and thousands of books fighting for shelf space, wasting precious paper, invading poor suckers' homes. People, especially fat people, will believe anything if they are desperate enough. They get set up for starvation, dream of success, and invite nothing but failure into their lives with these endlessly similar diets. Women end up fatter than ever, even more willing to settle. Why would I want to add my own words to this blizzard of diet/fitness crap?

So, I stay on the fence another day.

Yet, I keep the new folder marked "Tamara Hill" on my desktop. I stall. I'm busy. I have other deadlines. Another week goes by. My agent asks, "Have you spoken to her yet?" My magazine editor calls: "Oh, you really must call her. She's the next Susan Powter. Better yet, think Richard Simmons, but imagine a woman who is also a mother. I just know she is saying something very special. I love her."

I stare at the photos of this formerly obese woman who has transformed herself. She weighed 250 pounds and wore a size 24/26. I'm not sure that I like her, but my reaction is based on nothing tangible. Is it because I think she is just one more diet/fitness guru trying to cash in on women's distaste for their bodies? Perhaps. Visually, I soak up the new "Tamara"—100 pounds lighter and now a fitness phenomenon in her local Augusta, Georgia, community. Harrummph. Sounds a bit fanatical to me.

I dial the number, her number, finally, expecting (or perhaps even hoping) to speak to an answering machine. Suddenly, the strong, melodious, unstoppable voice on the phone takes me by complete, utter surprise. No, it's not her machine that has picked up my call, but I'm not disappointed. It's Tamara Hill, a thirty-eight-year-old mother of five, and you will soon want to know as much as you possibly can about her just as I did. With the untiring zeal of a fun-loving, excitable, yet exciting, missionary, she launches into stories, words of wisdom, bites of information, and the sound advice of a woman who has been there, done that, felt exactly that way: *fat!*

"Oh Lord, I was fat, Maryann. I was a fat gal, raised by a fat mom. Though I wasn't always fat as a child, I knew nothing about my body when I was growing up. I wasn't even told anything about menstruation. Looking back now, it's hard to believe that I ever let myself go so far. A second-generation descendant of Swedish, Norwegian, and Danish immigrants, I've always been tall and big-boned. Actually, when I was in high school, I was told that I had a nice figure. Like so many other women, I never had the weight problem until I started having my babies. Married at eighteen, I'm the mother of five and had my first at age nineteen. I was a full-time stay-at-home mom just like my mom, and for years, I concentrated on raising my kids and maintaining my home. And, just like my mother, I joined the 58 million obese people in the United States by gaining an average of 20 pounds with each of my pregnancies."

We are still on the phone an hour later. I am captivated by the sound of her voice, by her struggle, and by her spirit. She never misses a beat. After so many years of eating anything at all and all day long, moving as little as possible and growing fatter and fatter, she defined a mission that is almost incredible when you contrast it with her past. Here is a woman who was unhappily married, obese, and a home-day-care provider on a Southern army base just seven years ago. See her now, as I did in 1998: a motivational/fitness speaker, a local TV and radio guest, an AFAA step-certified instructor, a certified (NDEITA and ACE) primary aerobics instructor, an AEA water-certified exercise instructor, and the architect of a successful, hospital-based support and educational program called "Fat Chat with Tamara." Depending on the day of the week and the particular time of that day, you can find her at Aiken Regional Medical Centers in Aiken, South Carolina, at the Powerhouse Gym on Washington Road in Augusta, or way out in Edgefield, South Carolina, at Fitness Works. She is absolutely fascinating. Even if you have never wanted to lose more than ten pounds in your life, you fall in love with her message and want to know her story as well as her secrets. If you are an average American woman—and I am—the message is just too good to be true. I am quickly planning to go for a walk as soon as I hang up the phone. I've been sitting too long. Suddenly, I crave exercise.

"Your body is a marvelous piece of machinery. Nothing can duplicate it. No scientist and no inventor could ever come up with the human body," she tells me in this first lesson. I look down at my thighs. Oh, really. "There is nothing hideous or fearful about your body, but it will wear out if you carry an excess load of fat," she explains. Nothing complicated here, I think. Then, Tamara picks up steam . . . angry steam because she is furious with the multimillion-dollar diet and fitness industry as well as the media-made representation of the perfect woman. "She isn't a size 8 without a single ounce of flab. The average woman will never be that thin. She's shapely. She's soft. Thirty percent of her body is fat. Look at me," she says, and so I pick up the photo of Tamara that appeared in *McCall's* magazine. "This is what fit looks like. I'm thirty-seven inches on top. My waist is whooooaaaa maybe twenty-eight or twenty-nine inches. I weigh 150 to 155 pounds, and I'm only 5'7". I'm not 110 pounds, and I won't kill myself to weigh that or look like that perfect model on the cover of a fitness magazine."

Each runner has a different finish line—the goal each person has set.

DENNIS WAITLEY

What makes a critical difference here is her experience. Painful memories of being fat—yes, please say the word, *fat*—she insists, have set her apart from others preaching and teaching weight loss. "I am the average woman," she repeats, "and by sharing my own personal weight-loss story, I can motivate people and help them understand that fitness and good health are a matter of lifestyle. The sole purpose of Fat Chat is to motivate and inspire anyone who is overweight and unhealthy and not exercising regularly. I give support to anyone who has grown tired, frustrated, and discouraged and sees weight loss, weight maintenance, improved health, and exercising as things he or she will never be able to accomplish. It's all a matter of motivation. It's in your head.

"Seven years ago, I was back there. I had accepted that I was just going to be fat. I thought, 'I guess this is me.' I had always tried diets, mostly in secret—Slim Fast, Dexatrims, pills—starve and eat . . . starve and eat. I remember starving myself to the point where I would get up, be dizzy and nauseated, even black out. Those feelings are as clear as if it were just yesterday. For a while, I gave up and became comfortable with the idea of being fat."

I like her. You need her. I need her. I think we all need her. Picture me, still sitting in my third-floor home office in Upper Montclair, being pulled onto a path I had no intention of taking. She has that kind of power. The strength in her voice must be a mix of inspiration and optimism. In fact, optimism, as I understand it described by an anthropologist, is "the biology of hope." More phone minutes tick by. I don't want to leave her yet because I want to know the whole story of how she lost 100 pounds and transformed herself.

"Do you know that when you are obese, you don't believe anyone who is thin?" she says. "Fat people look at a thin person and think,

'Oh yeah, what do you know about moving my body? How do you know what it feels like to lift my legs? You don't know how badly my knees ache at the end of an evening or how my back hurts.' I would get into bed, and the fat would all fall around my heart and lungs, making it hard to breathe. I'd prop up the pillows. How can anyone who hasn't ever been fat know how that feels?" she asks.

> *The blows of life, the accumulation of difficulties, the multiplication of problems tend to sap energy and leave you spent and discouraged. In such a condition, the true status of your power is often obscured, and a person yields to a discouragement that is not justified by the facts. It is vitally essential to reappraise your personal assets.*
>
> Norman Vincent Peale,
> *The Power of Positive Thinking*

What she has learned are simple secrets everyone needs more than ever. We hang up that day determined to keep our chat sessions going and to meet as soon as possible. Her hometown. In the Powerhouse Gym. At the Aiken Regional Medical Centers. At Fitness Works. In my attic office. Across my kitchen table. In New York. Wherever . . . whenever we can talk, we talk.

In the pages to follow, using both of our voices, I will put you in the midst of some of Tamara's weekly Fat Chat programs. To make you feel even more at home, we will also share the words of letter writers—women just like you. What I want you to feel more than anything in the world is her spirit. Without it, these eight simple, personal secrets and one important step won't make any more sense to you than the diet book you bought last year (and never finished reading) or the program you dropped out of last month (after paying good money). Turn to Webster's dictionary and you'll see that *spirit* is "an animating or vital principle held to give life to physical organisms . . . the activating or essential principle influencing a person . . . the feeling, quality, or disposition characterizing something."

You can't buy spirit. Spirit is essential . . . the ultimate key to your success or failure.

Some people have the power to instill their spirit in others. They exude it and make the rest of us believe that all things are possible.

Let Tamara Hill get under your skin so she can give you a bit of her spirit.

Now let me take you to one of the places I visited in my quest to discover how she lost 100 pounds. (Ahem, her complete transformation was not, I repeat not, the result of a diet!)

The Program

Success comes in cans; failure comes in can'ts.

GOD'S LITTLE DEVOTIONAL HANDBOOK

Aiken Regional Medical Centers:

Take a long, deep breath. This isn't going to be difficult. I know because I was there and watched Tamara Hill in action.

Picture a hospital gymnasium and a circle of chairs. There are no mirror-lined walls in this setting. That would be too scary. It's a Tuesday evening, 6:45 and nearly time to begin. Eight to ten women, in all sizes and shapes and of all ages, are dressed comfortably in old leotards, shorts, baggy T-shirts, jeans. Some have come in straight-from-work clothes. Several—I'm in this category—have just finished an hour-long exercise class led by Tamara. A majority are obese. They have answered ads, read about Tamara in the local paper, picked up her story from a radio broadcast, or seen her on their local TV morning news. They have been looking for answers and have come to the right place—a refuge in a society that scorns and belittles women who are fat. This is the perfect setting in which to share successes, letdowns, recipes, concerns, questions, and fears. Want to know where to find something fat-free and sugar-free that will satisfy a chocolate craving? One of the participants, Linda, tells Ann, who has the hungry sweet tooth, "Look for Canfield's diet chocolate fudge soda. It's sugar-free and caffeine-free, too."

Sit down. You are among friends. You are welcome just the way you are. Relax. This is not a class in which you will be harshly judged. There are no failures here. You are not on an impossibly difficult journey. Do you brush your teeth every morning? Yes? Well, then, of course you can do this.

"To lose 100 pounds, you have to find the truth about the diet industry's losing game," Tamara explains. "You are a victim, or should I say casualty, of the $45 billion diet industry. This is a business, an ever-growing business, that wants your money. It has compounded your problem with fat. You are supposed to fail so you can come back and pay more money to lose the same weight you've already paid to get rid of. Come on, now, how much weight have you lost and gained in your life?" she asks.

Susann, Linda, Marcy, Rita, Wendy, and Jenny do some arithmetic. A chorus of "500 pounds," "140 pounds," "75 pounds," "60 or more pounds," "100 pounds," and "I have no idea but I'll guess 150 pounds," rings out in response. Now comes the sad kicker. "How much of the weight you lost have you regained?" Tamara asks. "Five hundred pounds," "140," "75," "100," "100 plus," and "150 plus more pounds," they answer in turn.

"Losing and gaining can be a vicious cycle until you eventually find yourself where I was: stuck and settling for an unhealthy life. Let's face it, because you are so vulnerable, you are being set up to be ripped off. Don't feel guilty. I was in the same place where you are," she explains. "Even if you do manage to succeed for a time by relying on the pills, supplements, shakes, or starvation, or the protein, pineapple, rice, soup, or grapefruit diets, you are no longer a profit-making piece of the big financial picture. That's why your success has to be short-lived. You and your diet dollars are needed to fuel profits. If you lose your excess weight once and for all, your business is also lost. The weight-loss industry is making a profit on your being fat and on your continuing struggle to get thinner. There are people you don't even know who have a stake in your staying fat."

Clearing away the guilt, she has climbed onto her soapbox, figuratively speaking, and while she may be pointing out issues that could already be apparent to some of us, her approach works wonderfully. Everyone in the room who has gained and lost the same weight year in and year out understands that dieting hasn't helped. In fact, restrictive diets have hurt them, emotionally and physically. We listen. We like what we hear. Blaming the diet industry feels so pleasant. A burden of guilt is lifted away.

"The diet industry thrives on what I like to call a three-easy-payment-plan mentality. Can't you just hear it on those television promos—the infomercials inviting you to buy the latest? Plunk your money down and in three, three . . . yes, three . . . easy payments, you too can wear a size 8 for your reunion, by Christmas, in time for bathing-suit season, or in seven days. The advertisements make promises these products can't possibly deliver. Yes, if you just make these three easy installments at their low, low price of $19.95 or whatever, you will be able to breathe away the excess weight. Yes, breathing away pounds has actually been a theory behind a bestselling book and program. Can you imagine? My God, you and I both know that it's not possible to breathe away obesity. Yet, haven't we tried?"

She mocks, "Do this simple exercise for just six minutes a day. Hah!

"Money-back guarantee if you don't lose. Right! Who ever gets a refund? Do you know anyone who has ever been granted her money back? I don't.

"You'll never sweat again. Short. Easy. Quick. Fast.

"Listen up," she tells the circle of women. "Do you realize that losing more than two or maybe three pounds of fat in a week is impossible? If the scale says that you've lost more than that, you aren't really losing excess fat. Don't believe me? Ask your doctor!"

The vast amount of money spent on diet clubs, special foods, and over-the-counter remedies, estimated to be on the order of $30 to $50 billion yearly, is wasted.

NEW ENGLAND JOURNAL OF MEDICINE

Tamara presses her case. "The diet industry is sickening because it is built upon both subtle and outright lies. It is sickening because success is based on an ideal that doesn't put good health first. It is sickening because it pushes women, children, and teens over the edge and into life-threatening eating disorders. I'm tellin' you that following someone else's diet plan or regimen won't get you where you need to be: in control over your own life. The diet industry robs you of your own power to decide what you want to eat, when you are going to eat it, how you are going to exercise."

Two seats away from me in the circle of chairs is a young woman who isn't convinced at all. Her frustration is palpable. She wants more structure. Tamara understands exactly where she is emotionally and mentally, and she steps into a new direction. "Everywhere I go, people want to know exactly what I eat," she says. " 'Give me the Tamara Hill diet,' they say, 'so I can eat what you eat and lose weight.' Well, I can tell you *exactly* what I eat, but how long do you think you'll be able to eat exactly what I eat? A week? Two weeks? A month? Not very long, I'd guess. You'll get tired of my favorite foods within a week or two. Oh sure, maybe you'll lose a pound or two or even more, but big deal. Will you be changing your own life for the better? I don't think so." She concludes, "Your plan—what you eat every day and how you move your body—has got to work for you, not me. It's got to be that way so you can keep on doing it and enjoying every step of your journey every day for the rest of your life. Habit, habit, habit . . . that is my message. Your name is not Jenny Craig, Susan Powter, or Richard Simmons. Their plans work for them, but in order for you to lose weight once and forever, your plan has to have your name and lifestyle on it. No one else's will work. This is the God's honest truth."

> *The restraints of a diet lead to a binge, regardless of the personality, character, or starting weight of the dieter. . . . Dieters are like tightly wound springs—the more restrained their eating, the tighter the spring. Once a dieter goes off his or her diet, the spring releases. The tighter that spring has been wound, the more forceful is its release. The more restrictive the diet, the bigger the binge.*
>
> JANE R. HIRSCHMANN AND
> CAROL H. MUNTER,
> *OVERCOMING OVEREATING*

"Just remember: If I can do it, so can you. I know how you feel, and I can help.

"The short, easy, quick, fast way to good health is a big, fat lie promoted by an industry that is making a huge profit on your being fat."

Nice. Nice. This feels very nice, as if a burden is being lifted. Blaming the diet industry is just so very perfect.

Tamara's Journey . . . in Her Own Words

> *It is good to have an end to journey towards; but it is the journey that matters in the end.*
>
> URSULA K. LEGUIN

At Her Kitchen Table on Linderwood Drive:

My mom grew up in an era when women didn't move much. Her thing was sitting and knitting, or sitting and sewing. As a child and young woman, she had been slender and beautiful. She was also smart. By the time she had me at age forty-two, she was 5'6" and 100 pounds overweight. I was the baby in my family; I have four brothers and two sisters, and I was born eight years after my youngest brother.

With my mother's obesity came related health problems. In her early fifties, she developed Type II diabetes which affected her body's ability to heal as well as her eyesight. Her health continued to go downhill, and pretty soon she was on dialysis for kidney failure. Finally, her heart showed the strain. Congestive heart failure ruined the final years of her life.

Meanwhile, my father was never fat. A hardworking construction guy, he could always eat whatever he wanted, and his body used up the food for fuel. His metabolism was like that. He had amazing energy, and I owe everything to him. There he was . . . a six-foot guy with a big, fat—really huge—wife, and he never wavered in his love for her. For the last three years of my mother's life, he was her nurse, and they traveled to various medical centers trying to find ways to get her well.

My mom didn't choose to be ill, but she was, and no one spoke about the F-A-T. No one ever talked about her problem. This includes my older siblings, who stepped cautiously away from the subject. Not even her doctors were clear or constructive with her about the fat. In fact, I didn't associate her various illnesses with her obesity at all. Oh, sure, one or another physician may have said to her, "Mrs. Peterson, you should lose weight," but no one went the extra mile to help her find out how and what she could do. No one said to her, "Are you exercising? What are you eating?" How she loved to eat! She baked for everyone in the family and ate for any reason. You know the pattern: she would eat if she was happy, sad, or confused. Eating was always the answer.

At her biggest, she hit almost 300 pounds and carried the extra weight mostly in her upper body. She didn't have hips like me, but she was big-boned like me, and we both have a dimple in our chins. No one else in my family has that dimple. Just me. And my mother. I used to be told, "You are the spittin' image of your mother." When I look at those old photos of her, I think, "Whooooaaa, that's me."

Yes, that tie to my mom is frightening, and yet, my mother's life and her death proved to be a catalyst for catastrophic change in my life.

Saying is one thing and doing is another.

MONTAIGNE

Seven years ago, when I was only thirty-two, I was in terrible shape. Not only did I weigh more than 250 pounds, but I also had undergone surgery for my gallbladder and for removal of ovarian cysts, as well as an appendectomy. I had high cholesterol and high blood sugar, an early sign of diabetes. Oh, I almost forgot to mention my asthma. I took my poor health for granted and never really associated my lack of energy with the fat. I felt normal and right in place with my friends and neighbors because many of them were obese, too.

Fat was common on the streets where I lived. Other women I knew were having babies, taking care of kids, and were just as heavy as I was or even heavier. My husband, now ex-husband, was stationed at Fort Jackson at the time, an army base in South Carolina.

I guess I just couldn't see myself clearly or where I was headed physically. Was I blind? Yes, emotionally speaking, I think I was. Sure, I looked in the mirror, but I don't think I wanted to see what I had become: *fat*! I know I didn't think I was *that big* because I distinctly remember the shock of catching a glimpse of myself in a car window when I was heading into the grocery store. *Could that big woman be me?* Sometimes when I was getting dressed in the morning and putting on my bra, I would look down and say to myself, "God, is this really my bra?" Yes, my bra was that big. Remember, I hadn't been a fat child, so the obesity crept up, and in my mind, I just couldn't possibly look quite that huge. I was definitely in denial.

Isn't it so true? You may be miserable when you are fat, but you don't want to think it's your fault. You see your weight as beyond your control. When you are more than 100 pounds overweight, you talk about diets and even try them. I know you do because I did, too. You look for all kinds of quick fixes.

I would dream of losing some weight, but I didn't make a clear connection between the fat and my poor health. Sure, sure, I wanted to lose weight, but that was so I could *look* good. You know, thinking back about those efforts, I know I didn't take them seriously. If I lost some pounds, that would be great, but if I didn't, so what. What was the big deal? I could always blame my failure on my aching feet, my busy day, my newest baby.

Somewhere along the way, I really gave up and got comfortable with the idea of being fat. I'd think, "Well, I guess this is just me." Why not? Isn't there a movement out there now to promote the rights of fat people who want to remain fat but gain more respect?

Fat gets in the way of reality. You just aren't in touch or able to think rationally because so much of your emotional health comes from food.

All this changed for me after my mother's death and her funeral on January 23, 1992. Traveling by car back to Minnesota where my family was gathered for the burial, I didn't in any way link my mom's obesity-related health problems to my own. I was sad, but she had been so sick for so long, and her death just didn't have anything to do with me . . . or so I thought. I couldn't possibly be in the same boat she had been in. I was huge but blamed my size on my metabolism, my genes, or anything but me. I was in that much denial. I didn't care about my cholesterol level. I didn't even know my blood sugar level, and though I was tired all the time, I didn't think, "I'd have more energy if I lost weight."

Fat was beside the point. This was just who I was: a soldier's wife, a mother of five, a busy home-day-care provider with no time to think, let alone care, about my own needs.

For God's sake, I didn't care about my own health, and I was attending the funeral of my own mother who had just died of obesity-related complications. I was obese, too. I hadn't even brought a dress to wear because I could find nothing suitable that fit me. After driving all the way to Elk River, Minnesota, I had to go downtown to the local fat ladies' store and try on a zillion different outfits. The dress I finally chose was hideous and size 24/26.

We make our decisions and then our decisions turn around and make us.

F. W. Boreham

When my siblings saw me the day before the service, they were surprised. I hadn't been home in quite some time, and though they had heard I'd gained weight, the reality of me was pretty powerful. Funny, but none of them are obese. Just me. Just like mom.

My father could hardly bear the sight of me. I made him sick. Having cared for my mother for so long, he looked at me and felt real pain. Every time he glanced in my direction, he saw my mother, the fat woman he had loved and lost. The fat had killed her, and there I was: his baby daughter, just as fat. Later in my parents' home after the funeral, he let me feel the brunt of all the emotions he had tried to suppress. Fear, anger, and disappointment came pouring out. He wasn't trying to be mean. I know that. His unplanned words flowed straight from his heart. Despite all that, I didn't want to hear him and can remember thinking, "How can he be so cruel to me?"

"You are going to end up just like your mother," he said with tears streaming down his cheeks. We were both crying.

"Stop it, Dad. Not now," I begged him. He couldn't.

"This fat. This fat will kill you. Do you want that? Do you think I like seeing you this way?"

Then, he tossed my mother's diabetes sugar-testing kit at me. "Here, you are going to need this. Keep on going the way you are headed, and you'll need it very soon. Then, who's going to take care of you?"

On the long trip back to Fort Jackson, his words stayed with me. I couldn't erase the tape playing them in my head. Believe me, I tried. The crying, the arguing, the turmoil of a night spent without sound sleep had been awful. I was mad at my dad and continued to blame everybody and anybody but myself. I didn't even call him for weeks afterward. Can you imagine how awful that was . . . for both of us?

My poppa saved my life. I know it. I am 110 percent certain that without his outbursts of loving concern, I would have left that funeral and not changed a thing in my life. I would have ended up with a stroke or a heart attack or diabetes. My poppa made me think, and slowly . . . slowly . . . slowly, the cogs began turning in my brain.

Whoooaaa. One of the first things I did when I got home is not what you may be thinking. No, I didn't start eating right, exercising, or checking my blood sugar levels. In fact, just the opposite: I hid the sugar-testing kit in our hall closet.

Breathlessly, I filled my cart with boxed desserts, canned potato sticks, whatever crossed my path. Wheeling past the delicatessen counter, the red center of a roast beef caught my eye, "I'll take that," I said . . . "Lady, this piece of beef runs a good 18, 19 pounds. It'll cost you about 40 bucks." . . . I was some anonymous eccentric fat lady. "That's my business," I snapped.

WALLY LAMB, *SHE'S COME UNDONE*

2

To Lose 100 Pounds . . .

"I Became Accountable to Me and Only Me"

The Person

When you have to make a choice and you don't make it, that is in itself a choice.

WILLIAM JAMES

A School in Suburban Augusta:

Thursday, midmorning, the front-office lobby of an Augusta middle school is a busy place to be. Parents arrive for appointments with teachers or school counselors. Phones are ringing behind a chest-high counter. Teachers, school administrators, and secretaries buzz in and out. A few sixth-, seventh-, and eighth-grade students stand about. Tamara and I have arrived together on a sunny September day. Dressed in a nifty green and black exercise outfit, Tamara is waiting to meet the chair of the physical education department, who has arranged for her to speak to 200 students now assembling on bleachers in the gym down the hall. She is holding a large poster prominently featuring before-and-after photographs of herself. The before shots are pretty dramatic.

The curiosity behind the counter starts to build. Two secretaries can't take their eyes off the poster. "Is that you?" one asks. All around us, there is a chorus of ooohs and wows. From around an open door, several other adults now emerge from back offices. One of the women is very obese. "How did you do it? Why did you do it?" she asks Tamara, leaning forward, visibly hungry for answers.

Tamara's response shocks me. As a motivational speaker, she rarely uses negative lines of thought. In fact, I generally find her approach to be the kinder, gentler variety. Yet, in the spotlight there in this crowded school waiting room, she looks straight at this inquiring woman and replies in a strong, loud, clear voice, "Because fat kills!"

After a deliberate pause, she adds softly, "I can say this because I've been there. I know how you feel, and I've earned the right to speak so freely. I know what fat feels like and how dangerous it is for your health."

I'm thinking that this curious school secretary is going to shrink up emotionally and scuttle away in anger. Wouldn't you agree with me? However, that doesn't happen at all. She looks right back at Tamara and is buoyed by her directness. She's not offended at all, and like a kindred spirit, she says, "Next time, speak to the adults here, not just the kids."

"Oh girl, you bet I will," Tamara says sweetly. "Call me and I'll come."

Whew. Tamara Hill has this way of becoming immediately intimate with the people she touches. Nothing threatening here! If I called someone I had just met "girl," after telling her that fat was going to kill her if she didn't change her ways, I'd be making an instant enemy. My high-energy, softhearted coauthor does no such thing. Like a missionary with the emotional touch of a Midas or a Pied Piper promoting healthy habits of living, she manages to make people want to join her.

"I want to be a role model and inspiration for others who want to achieve a healthier lifestyle," she says. "I have decided that this is something I must do for life. I am committed to this forever. I am a woman with a mission to take a proactive stance instead of a reactive stance toward health and wellness in my own life, in my children's lives, in the lives of the people I meet. I'm nobody special."

To the small audience there in the reception area, this last statement doesn't ring true. She is very special, and in action, she is hardly just anybody. As heads turn and a line of secretaries follow us through the crowds of kids in the hallway and down the gym, the electricity in the air around her is saying something else entirely. The chair of the physical education department, a small, strong, compact woman, leads the way, telling Tamara, "I'm so glad you are here. The kids can't wait!"

The Program

Your past is the one part of your life over which you have absolutely no control. No amount of remorse, regret, or bad feeling will change history. You do, however, have control over your present and your future.

MICHAEL LEBOEUF, *IMAGINEERING*

A Baptist Church Somewhere in Georgia:

The minister has enlisted Tamara to help kick off a sixteen-week Bible-study program called First Place which is designed to encourage his older congregation to get healthier as they learn. About twenty-five people have gathered at noontime to hear her speak. "It's my attitude," she says. "That's what they say about me. When the lady from the church called to invite me, she said, 'Oh Tamara, you are just so energetic, and I know this is the attitude we need to get our people geared up and going.'"

No one in the audience looks as excited as Tamara at first. Bright-eyed, posture-perfect, parading back and forth across the front of the room and down the aisles, pretty soon, she launches into the kind of emotion-laden logic that changes lives. If they have come only for the free lunch, these church members soon realize that they are being offered much more.

"Obesity in your families?" she asks. Look around the crowd and you can guess the answer is positive for the majority. "I know. I know," she says. Her "I was a fat gal raised by a fat mom" line gets nods of immediate approval. The audience relates. Everyone has obesity in the family. She points to the image of her fat self on her poster. "The lesson I learned from my momma was to find a husband, get married, have babies, and take care of my family. This was clear for me. This is what I did for so many years: I did for my husband. I did for my kids. I did for my community. There was no me; there just wasn't any time for me. Maybe I thought about doing something for me, but then I'd just say, 'Forget it.' I had no time and no energy. Only later in my life did I realize that I have to be me before I can be anybody for anyone else."

She points to her poster again and insists, "This was me, not taking any interest in me. My weight was up over 250. My cholesterol was 268. My blood sugar was over 160." People in the audience are nodding. They know her so well. She can get inside their heads and their hearts. "Now this is me, seven years later, taking an interest in myself," she says, pressing both hands to her chest. She twirls around, standing tall. "You know, this is the only body I've got. This is my heart," she says. "This is my soul and my mind. I have to sacrifice in other areas of my life because I need to take care of my health.

"How many people here have diabetes?" Hands go up.

"How many people here have other health concerns like high blood pressure or heart disease?" More hands go up. One woman raises her hand and says, "My doctor says I have high cholesterol but that it's hereditary."

"Oh thank you, Jesus," Tamara says, but there is no sense of reproach in her voice, and the fresh-faced, fifty-something questioner is not frightened into submission. Everyone laughs. "This is just great," Tamara tells her. People feel comfortable. You can see other hands reaching up into the air as people get ready to speak out. "So high cholesterol in your family! Do you know what? I don't care if these things have been in your family for generations. You still have control over your body. You still have choices. In fact, because your doctor says you've got some kind of hereditary health problem, you have even more of a reason to be making good choices. What are you doing every day? Are you moving your body? Every time you put food into your mouth, you are making a choice that will have consequences. Some choices have important, positive benefits for your health. Others have negative consequences. It's up to you."

From the back of the crowd, someone says, "Yeah, well, I've got diabetes and there's nothing I can do about it."

Tamara quickly answers, "I'll bet you that it's not Type I diabetes but Type II."

"How did you know that?"

The facts, she demonstrates, are eye-opening. "Only 700,000 to 800,000 people are diagnosed as Type I diabetics, whereas there are more than 10 million with Type II, a disease that threatens all of us, especially once we reach our fifties. There are two basic things that can bring on Type II diabetes: not eating right and a sedentary lifestyle. Am I right? You bet I'm right. All of us . . . you and me both . . . many, many of us have total, total control over these aspects of our lives, don't we?

"For God's sake, it's high time we redefined what is health and what is fit here in the United States. For years, all of our efforts have been on 'how we look' and 'looking good.' Do you realize that it wasn't until I stopped concentrating on 'looking good' and put all my efforts toward wellness and health that I started feeling better emotionally and physically? I gained more energy and was finally able to lose those 100 pounds.

"Bodies come in all shapes and forms and sizes, and we should be darn proud of the one we've got. Fitness is possible for people of all abilities, ages, and personalities. Fitness, in fact, has nothing to do with those three numbers on the scale that so many of you focus on every morning and every night."

Love yourself first and then everything else falls in line.

LUCILLE BALL

She announces, "Number one issue here is that you can't be accountable to a scale. What you weigh is not a good measure of your health. You can't be accountable to some doctor's sheet of paper, either. Are you going to let some insurance company tell you that according to your height, your weight has got to be yadda, yadda, yadda?" she says, singsonging her way into this audience's heart. "Just say to yourself right now: 'I'm not even going to worry about what I weigh. I am not going to worry about those numbers on the scale.' Those three numbers are not a true indication of your state of health. At 5'7" and

150-some pounds, I'm off those charts, but I'm fit. I'm healthy." She adds, "If I can do it, so can you!

"Ask yourself: Am I moving my body? Am I eating pretty much what I ought to be eating? Do I have energy?"

"This is a long process. I'm going to help you. I'm going to bring these issues to light so you can get to the end of the tunnel." People are smiling. The minister is happy. Though stomachs may have begun to growl with anticipation of the arrival of lunch at the back of the hall, Tamara continues to talk about nutrition, exercise, and power. One lady says, "Ms. Hill, I just don't have any willpower."

"Pshaw," Tamara answers. "Let's not even talk about willpower here today. Let's talk about people who have set you up to fail. Let's talk about feelings of guilt and depression and desperation. You have given your power to others who are making you feel like a failure. You look at those exercise ladies in their size-2 spandex leotards, and no wonder you think, 'I can't do what she is doing.' Or, you see only those three numbers on the scale and a doctor wagging his finger at you, or your medical chart. You are not being accountable to you, and only you. You need to be empowered with positive thoughts, positive feelings. It's got to be positive, or it won't work.

"No, no, no," she repeats to the beaming woman who is primed to start her own journey to wellness but worried about willpower. "I am not going to feed you negative feelings or anxieties. It's really just common sense. I work at what I do. Good health doesn't come in a bottle, magic potion, or lotion, but isn't yours worth working for? Believe me when I tell you that you have the power—all the power you need to do this is right inside yourself."

Most powerful is he who has himself in his own power.

SENECA

It's lunchtime. You can smell the chicken. Everyone in the congregation waits to see what Tamara will choose from the buffet line. Will it be the fatty fried version or the plain grilled? The green beans? The potatoes? "For God's sake," she says afterward. "Jeeeez, I don't promote thinness; I just promote health. And I do eat fried chicken . . .

just not every day and in excess quantities. I took off some of the skin, but I'm tellin' you: I'm living proof that my program works. Every week at various weight-loss clinics and obesity centers, people climb onto scales, look at those numbers, and become more accountable to them than anything or anyone else. I know it. Everyone who has ever dieted needs to know it, too. You can't experience success when you are empowered by depression, desperation, or shame or when someone else is in charge."

The rapture of pursuing is the prize.

HENRY WADSWORTH LONGFELLOW

Tamara's Journey . . . in Her Own Words

At My Kitchen Table in Montclair, New Jersey:

Let me take you back to me, about eight years ago. I try not to remember or dwell on those days, but you need to know what happened and how I began to emerge. I want my story to make a difference. I am a butterfly now. Once upon a time, I was this fat, chunky caterpillar, and of course, no one could see my beauty. I had spun a cocoon from which I would eventually emerge. My whole world has opened up. My self-esteem is a mile high, and my outlook has changed 100 percent. The difference in me is profound. When I walk down the street, I hold my head up. With my chin up, what people notice is not my size but my stature. I'm not skinny, and I never will be.

> *Oscar de la Renta, the fashion designer, insists that what makes a woman glamorous in one of his dresses is her sense of self. That comes "from within," he explains. Take two women in the same dress, and the more glamorous one will not be the thinner one but the woman who is more positive from the inside out.*

Oh Lord, nowadays I make full eye contact with people I meet whereas before, my shoulders were hunched over and my head was down. When I enter a room, I'm upbeat, and I know that others sense this. Yes, my size has changed, but that's almost a side effect of what was even more important in taking me from back there to where I am now.

My life used to be depressing. Working as a licensed home-day-care provider at Fort Jackson, I had my own five kids, but I also took care of five or six more children nearly every day. Don't get me wrong: I like kids. I've always liked them. I still do. I'm a good mom. My husband was a soldier, and providing for our large family on a military paycheck wasn't easy. We needed the money I could make in my day-care business. You can imagine.

The alarm would go off at 5:30 or 6 A.M. My youngest, Cassandra, was just a baby then. I was at my heaviest when she was about eight months old. Isn't it so true? You do what you have to do—for others, but most of the time, you pay little regard to your own needs. Military wives are like so many other women and mothers everywhere. I meet them all the time. Days can be long, with rarely a break. My energy level was rock-bottom. Excitement in my life? Hah! Where? When?!

My husband would leave the house for his early-morning PT, which stands for "physical training." This was the army, and those guys have to stay in shape, so there were gyms located all over the base. He'd head for the gym about 6 A.M. At this point, exercise was not on my to-do list. Moving my body was difficult, so I didn't do it much. My muscles were buried beneath layers of fat and had been for years.

Meanwhile, back in my bedroom, *my* itinerary would be more like: get up, get dressed, get the kids ready before more kids arrive. OK, so after I dragged myself out of bed, the first thing I'd have to face was the clothes question. What was in my closet? Ugh. Nothing worth remembering, that's for sure. My pants were just enormous. I was a size 24 or 26, as I mentioned before, and even those got snug; I could barely zip them up. You kid yourself about how you look when you are that big.

Parents would drop kids off early on their way to work. On Fort Jackson and on any army post, child-care providers are monitored and certified. Officially, the army allows certified providers to care for up to ten or eleven kids at one time, but that number includes your own children. I always cared for another baby about the same age as Cassandra as well as two or three toddlers in my daughter Kaye's age range.

My older two boys would be off to school for the day. There are twelve years between my oldest and youngest.

There's a routine and a daily plan you follow. I'd have a special time for breakfast, followed by midmorning snacks, some activities, lunch, a trip outside, more snacks, naps, and a regular predictable pattern for the kids every day—and for me. I'd make peanut butter and jelly sandwiches and eat one for every one I handed out. Cakes, desserts, and lots of sugar sodas were always on hand. I'd buy those big sixteen-ounce glass bottles. Had to have lots of sugar soda. That's what we call it here in the South.

I'm tellin' you, I was this big fat momma, right in the middle of lots of little kids all day long. The kids were never the problem, however. The problem was me. But you've got to remember: I wasn't out of the ordinary. Many of my friends were fat, too.

I didn't care about myself, or perhaps I should say that I didn't make time to care about myself. Who was I trying to impress? Where was I going each day? Nowhere. The center of my life was my home and, more to the point, my kitchen. I didn't even talk to adults very much during the day. Surrounded by preschoolers, I simply had no thoughts of going anywhere. It wasn't that I was unhappy; it was just how my life was. Besides, I think I fed all my emotions with food. Around my neighborhood, other gals, fat gals, were doing the same thing. Our lives revolved around food, from those first trips to the kitchen to prepare breakfast right through to the last snack before turning in.

Isn't it so true? We are such creatures of habit. There I was in my house doing nothing for myself. I ate everything the kids couldn't finish, and I liked the fact that they were all so little because they were nonjudgmental. I was able to eat what I wanted without the fear of someone's making a snide comment or reproach. Never did I hear, "Are you sure you want to eat that?" Secretly, I was pleased with this fact of life. Then again, when I think back, I do recall trying to hide my treats from the kids on occasion, especially if I didn't want to share with so many. If I were eating ice cream or doughnuts, let's say, I'd shove the empty package to the bottom of the kitchen trash can.

Who was I foolin'? This kind of behavior just amazes me now. When I hid the remnants of those binges, I was certainly not being accountable to me and only me. I was more concerned with what other people, even little people, might think or say. There I was: huge, always exhausted, in poor health, and unable to blame my behavior on my own habits. I kept right on eating and never wanted to associate the consequences of my actions with me and my fat.

Isn't it so true that you might think about losing weight but never connect the weight to your high cholesterol or out-of-control blood sugar levels? When you are really obese, you don't want to think about your health. I think it is that simple. The rationale is that losing weight has nothing to do with saving your life; medicine and doctors are supposed to do that. I know that, for me, on the days when the numbers were higher than ever, I'd want to eat even more. Deep, deep denial is what this state of mind is called.

Habit is overcome by habit.

THOMAS Á KEMPIS

Oh, did I tell you that my ex-husband liked me fat? He was a stocky guy, who had been trained as a chef and whose own mother was big. So, I was just a big, safe gal for him. When I met him, I was already divorced with two children and 30 to 40 pounds overweight. I recall thinking, "Oh, I'm so lucky that this guy is paying any attention to me." I had no self-esteem, and he was a very controlling person: an awful combination. I will say, however, that he was never verbally abusive about my weight. Unlike many of the thousands of women who have written to me describing abusive relationships, my husband never subjected me to that kind of emotional trauma. Thank God no one ever made pig noises at me.

Within days after I arrived home from my mother's funeral, I let my life slip right back into its rutted routine. Where was my father's voice of reason? Drowned down to a whisper, that's where it went. I didn't want to think about my mother's death. I didn't want to bring back what my poppa had said. The sugar-testing kit was shoved out of sight in the back of the closet.

Yet, I just didn't feel very good and started to feel even worse in the weeks after Mom's death. At first, I tried to blame it on the psychological upset. Then, chest pains and headaches sent me to the army hospital's emergency room one day. My blood pressure was way up there, probably 140 over who knows what. Normal is 120 over 80, and I was certainly way above that. My pulse was racing at 118, when a normal pulse is 78 to 100. I was given an EKG (electrocardiogram), and the results were normal. I do have a history of a heart murmur, but that didn't seem to be the problem. The emergency physician's words are loud and clear in my memory: "Well, Mrs. Hill," he said, and not in a mean way, "the truth is: if you would get some of this weight off, you'd feel better and your blood pressure would go down."

Slam. Damn. He was a nice man, but I sat there steaming, fuming, and stuck in the same old don't-tell-me-what-to-do, I'll-eat-what-I-please place. Yadda. Yadda. Yadda. I was sent home from the hospital with the exact prediction my father had been trying to get into my head: The fat . . . the fat was going to kill me.

Though I had gone to the hospital that day looking for an excuse for my aches and pains, searching for someone or something else to blame, I came away with a hard lesson once again: The only person responsible for me and my health was me.

Now, here's the really scary part: One morning after my trip to the ER, I pulled the sugar-testing kit out from its hiding place. Having grown up with my mother's diabetes, I needed no instructions on exactly what to do with it. I had watched my momma test herself from the time I was a baby. She had suffered with Type II diabetes for more than twenty years. I also knew what this disease could do to a body. I poked myself to draw blood and then jotted down the number I had come up with: more than 160. Normal is anywhere from 70 to 120, and I was borderline diabetic, but I simply said to myself, "It'll go down tomorrow." For several days in a row, I repeated the test, but those numbers never went down. Though I recall thinking, "Jeez, this isn't good," I wasn't prepared to do anything about it . . . yet.

One evening, my neighbor, who wasn't quite as fat as me, stopped by to ask if I wanted to go to a Weight Watchers meeting with her. My initial response was almost a knee-jerk "No." But I stopped myself from adopting that so-you-think-I'm-too-fat defense mode and said, "Maybe." After all, she was a friend, a fellow home-day-care provider, and was only trying to help herself as well as me.

I was thirty-two years old when the two of us drove together to that first meeting in Columbia, South Carolina. Though the ride was only fifteen minutes, the most important journey of my life had begun. I signed in, waited in line to weigh in, and tried to put my head and heart right there. Yet, something inside me was still missing.

To Lose 100 Pounds . . .

"I Simply Started Moving"

The Person

Packing My Suitcase on a Sunday in September, 1998:

Tamara has forwarded along a copy of *Ms. Fitness* magazine that features an article about her remarkable transformation as well as an update on her current exercise schedule. I'm in awe of how much this woman moves her body day in and day out. Look at this routine and tell me that you wouldn't be as worried as I am:

- Aerobics/Step Aerobics—60 minutes, 5 times a week
- Run/Walk—60 minutes, 2 times a week
- Weight training—60 minutes, 2 or 3 times a week

It is late September as I pack to head off to Augusta where I'll be spending time following her around and taking as many classes and Fat Chat sessions as I possibly can. Just adding up the minutes she spends exercising makes me feel tired. Could this schedule be possible? Was the author of the article exaggerating the daily intensity with which Tamara attacks her new life . . . just a bit? Please God, will I make it through the next week in one piece? More important, is she obsessed with exercise?

"Oh girl, don't you worry," she tells me on the phone. "You'll be just fine. When I was heavy, if you had asked me about exercise, I would have answered, 'Ugghhh, I hate it.' I think I hated it because exercise, as it is presented on television and in magazines and infomercials, is horrible. Now I have a different mind-set. I love it. I'm teaching class and working as a personal trainer, which is why those minutes add up. As I became familiar with my body and how it moved five, six, seven years ago, I'd suffer—ooooohhh, did I hurt—but I knew it was just my body's way of saying, 'Hey, you've been neglecting me too long.' I never thought of giving up because deep down, I knew that moving my body was just great. I'm not that *Cosmo* woman; I'm almost forty, and I've got five kids. Hey, in answer to your question, 'Am I obsessed?' No, I am not obsessed. I've just built all this movement into my everyday life."

The good news is that it's never too late to begin an exercise program . . . even people in their seventies gained muscle and stamina on a regular program that included working with weights. Some felt so much better, they even abandoned their canes and walkers.

CHERYL HARTSOUGH,
The Anti-Cellulite Diet

The next day in the airport, I begin to experience the "everyday life" Tamara describes so enthusiastically. I'm sweating even before I step into the first of many aerobic workouts. The average daily temperature in Georgia in the fall is a lot hotter than in New Jersey. That and the humidity are factors I neglected to consider seriously when packing on Sunday. Cotton comfort clothes are essential around here.

In fact, what you must have if you are going to slip into Tamara Hill's lifestyle are lots of warm-weather exercise outfits. Nothing fancy is needed. Simple shorts, T-shirts, sweat socks, and sneakers are gear enough to get you through her day. No spandex. No glittery leggings. No tube tops. Just you feeling comfortable. From early morning when she wakes her children and makes sure book bags are packed, school buses are caught, and household essentials are covered until late in the evening when she finishes up a Fat Chat session or step aerobics class, Tamara is at ease and in clothes that allow her body to move.

"There aren't enough choices in exercise clothing for fat people," she insists. "Women need cotton, and they need to let the air reach their skin. If you cover up too much, your sweat isn't able to dissipate. When you exercise, it's a proven fact that your core body temperature will rise two to three degrees. So, if your normal temperature is 98.6 degrees Fahrenheit, then you are going to end up at least 100.8 or 101.8, and that's high. Your sweat means that your body's cooling system is working. The worst thing you can do is to prevent that sweat from being absorbed into cotton clothing or dissipated right off the skin's surface. Sweating is so neat and so healthy. I tell people who come to my classes bogged down in long pants and turtlenecked up tight that their bodies need to be able to cool off. Sweat can't escape if you are too covered up. You've got to get into shorts to release the moisture.

"Don't you know that those plastic suits are terrible?" she says definitively, referring to polyester warm-up suits. She's on a roll and such fun to follow. "Why do you think that runners in New York will shed their clothing in the dead of a cold winter? At the finish line of a marathon, if they don't put on additional clothing immediately, they'll get chilled. Sometimes after the twenty-six-mile race, for instance, you'll see runners putting on capes or stocking caps right away."

We are in her van, heading toward Aiken, South Carolina, for an evening exercise class, to be followed by a Fat Chat session. Tamara makes moving your body sound simple: "Almost anybody can walk. I always say to beginners—old, young, unfit, no matter where they are—that it takes very little coordination to walk. You may have to crawl before you can walk, but that's how I started. I can remember when I could walk only a quarter of a mile. I'd be walking with my ex-husband, with kids in the stroller. Basically, he'd push the stroller at first, and I kind of hung on. It was difficult for me to move my big legs." Looking at her now in the car, with her well-muscled but shapely legs in shorts, I try to visualize the "before" version of Tamara. It's not easy to do.

"These legs have come a long way from the big stovepipes I once had," she acknowledges. "I'm not saying mine are in Cindy Crawford's league, but I think I have wonderful legs now. I never want to compare myself with a model. My legs aren't skinny, but they are strong and sculpted. I used to have legs that were big and weak, and because of that, I had lower-back pain, knee problems, and shinsplints. There was no muscle strength in the quadriceps or my hamstrings.

"I've read and read and read and done a lot of research. I know what I'm talking about now. I've been studying this stuff for years now, taking courses and passing certification exams. It has taken me a lot of time, but I really want people to understand how movement can give them so much benefit in terms of muscular and skeletal fitness." She is exuberant and into her subject with a missionary zeal. Tamara's enthusiasm makes me sit up straighter in the front seat. Suddenly with shoulders aligned, I can breathe better, and the knot in my back isn't as tight.

We have 40 million reasons for failure, but not a single excuse.

RUDYARD KIPLING

She continues, "In class, you'll see that I always talk about how wonderful the human body is. I try to get my people to start thinking of their own bodies as tremendous and not something hideous or to be afraid of. So many women want to hide their bodies. They think of themselves as awful, when the truth is so far from that. I'll ask: 'How do you think your heart feels? Think about how hard your body must work to carry the extra fat?' I have this gift of connecting with them because I've been there. I know what it feels like to wear a 24/26. I remember what it was like to start moving, to have to push my body so hard that I would be in pain, not just physical pain but emotional as well. People would stare at me, and I'd be thinking, 'Oh God, how I must look.' Yet, I kept right on going. I think my compassion for others now springs from those experiences."

Exercise influences what you choose to eat because it depletes your limited carbohydrate stores. You'll actually crave fruit rather than fat.

ROBERT PRITIKIN, *Bottom Line* NEWSLETTER

The ride from Augusta to her evening's workplace is at least thirty minutes, and the back of her van is filled with the parts and parcels of her movable professional life: boxes of xeroxed handouts for class, exercise gear, her before-and after-posters, changes of clothing, bottles of water, and paperwork from Powerhouse Gym where she has been busy working as a personal trainer and selling memberships.

"I'm not a physician," she says insistently. "I don't have a degree. I'm not a dietitian. Yet, through me, others can understand that you don't have to be an expert to change your life. You just need to take an interest in your own body. Whatever is out there, read it, listen to the experts, experience movement, try, try, try, and then combine what you learn about yourself to create your own program. Maybe you can apply a little of this or a little of that and modify whatever you try.

"You need to work out a program that is just for you. I bring forth information and diet systems and pieces of equipment, and in class, I pose questions to get people to 'Love Self, Think Health, and Move It to Lose It!' Those are my three basic principles. The keys are regular exercise, eating sensibly, and being good to yourself . . . not just for a month or this year, but a regimen for life. We have total control over what we put into our bodies and how we exercise. You've got to take care of you and feed your mind with good stuff. No one else can do it for you."

Pulling up to the Aurora Pavilion at Aiken Regional Medical Centers, she races around to the back of the van, and together, we carry in this evening's paraphernalia. "Don't forget your shorts," she says to me. "You can change inside." Though I have long since rolled up my New York black suit jacket and shoved it into a carry-on bag, I'm in a skirt, straight from the airport and eager to start moving into her busy life. Yes, I'm still sweating.

Dr. Steven Blair, director of research and epidemiology at the Cooper Institute of Aerobics Research in Dallas, quotes a Scottish researcher's estimate that in Britain, average energy expenditures have dropped by 800 calories a day in the last twenty-five years. If anything, the decline has been even more precipitous on this side of the Atlantic. Even if you used just 100 calories a day less and ate the same amount, you would gain about ten pounds a year, nearly all of them as body fat, unless you are physically active.

JANE E. BRODY, *NEW YORK TIMES*

The Program

Inside the Aurora Pavilion at Aiken Regional Medical Centers:

Optimism is a tonic. Pessimism is a poison. Admittedly, everyone must be realistic. You must gather facts, analyze them candidly, and then strive to draw logical conclusions.

B. B. FORBES, *FORBES* MAGAZINE

Listen for just a minute to some of the voices I found in the pink-walled Aurora Pavilion later after exercise classes and during a Fat Chat session. They will help you sense the tone of this program. There is no lockstep approach to weight loss or rigid plan to follow for a definitive period of weeks. Yet, lessons are being learned and habits are being changed. Go back there with me. If you want to lose 20, 40, 80, 100 pounds or even more, you need to put your mind in shape first.

About 7 P.M., a polite quiet settles over the circle of women seated in folding chairs. "You don't know how difficult it was to ask someone in the hall for directions to this group," someone says. "I hate to say the word *fat*."

"Oh heck, why not say it?" an outspoken participant chimes in. "Tamara tells us to say the word *fat* out loud." A local newspaper reporter named Sharon Taylor has come to find out about the group for an article. Tamara, still buzzing by the hospital's main entrance, is awaiting stragglers. She doesn't want anyone getting lost or feeling less than loved this evening. "Sharing and caring," she insists, "that's what this is all about." Meanwhile, Sharon asks the group, "What does Tamara do that helps you stay motivated?" Their eagerness to share overtakes any lingering shyness about being in the company of two strangers. Instantly, answers pour out.

- "She lets us know that it's OK to be fat . . . as long as you are healthy."
- "Her spirit is contagious. She reminds me of the new minister at my church who is deliriously happy all the time."
- "Exercise makes me feel good, and Tamara says it changes my brain chemistry. I do get depressed as well as obsessed, so I need to come here."

- "I've got boobs. I've got hips, and Tamara makes me know deep down that this is wonderful."
- "I could feel stronger the very next week after I started weight training with Tamara."
- "I know that I can have success no matter what the scale says."
- "Those three numbers mean absolutely nothing."
- "Sometimes, it's hard not to give in to those diet ads all over the place. I looked at a product in the store recently, and the only thing that stopped me from buying the box was my thinking about what this group would say to me if I tried another quick fix."
- "Oh yeah, I know just what you mean. I put some quickie diet thing in my cart the other day and actually went up and down two or three more aisles before I looked at it and thought, 'What would Tamara say about this?' It was as if she were right there in the store with me."
- "Sometimes I come here thinking all the while, 'I don't want to be here. My wagon is really draggin'. By the time I leave, I'm full of energy."
- "I don't know exactly what it is, but I do know that there is something mental going on."
- "I didn't like to exercise. I didn't like it at all when I got started. But I've learned to like it. It's kind of like sex: I learned to like it, and I'm not lying."

With laughs all around, someone quickly counters, "Do you mean the exercise part or the sex part?"

Finally, before the laughter dies down, Tamara races in, sits down, and with a wide, kind of sly and happy glance around the circle, calls out, "Hey, how are you? Are you happy?"

"OK, listen up," she says. "Most of the women who write, call, and E-mail me have given up hope. I do get some letters from men, but it's the women like myself and like you gals who are most beaten down by failure and by this body-image thing. They are desperate and depressed about ever losing weight, and this kind of totally negative mind-set works against any real progress. Buulllliieeeeve me, if you've got an overwhelming focus on food and those pounds on the scale, then your head is in the wrong place. It's movement that counts the most . . . just a little bit and a little bit more every day," she tells us.

"Just get up. Don't even worry about all those experts tellin' you that you've got to get your heart up to some gol' darn target range for twenty to thirty minutes so many times a week."

Talk turns to dog walking, leaf raking, gardening, and biking to bakeries in Germany—a story Tamara promises to share. "You don't need to be obsessed or fanatical about this exercise deal. You just have to incorporate more movement into your lifestyle. Look at me," she says. "I move around a lot now, teaching five days a week, trying to do a little weight training on Saturdays and working as a personal trainer. This kind of activity makes it easy for me to sit down at the dinner table and eat more than you without gaining any weight. Want to know why?" she ask the puzzled group.

"'Cause I've got more muscle than you do. If there is a miracle, this is it: Muscle weighs more than fat and is more compact. Muscular women may weigh more but look smaller. I can wear a size 10 and weigh 150 pounds because of muscle." She rolls up the sleeve of her T-shirt and makes a muscle to show off her arm. "Isn't this amazing? Think about what my arms used to look like. Now, someone who has more fat than lean muscle could easily weigh less than 150 and not be able to squeeze into a 10.

"Those height/weight charts published by insurance companies and distributed in doctors' offices and diet centers have got it wrong," she asserts, "because the charts don't take body composition into consideration. The more muscle you have, the more you can eat. For every pound of muscle, you need thirty-five to fifty calories to make that muscle function. The reason your metabolism falls is that fat just sits there doing nothing metabolically. Muscle burns calories even when you are sleeping. And when you exercise or move your body even a little, your metabolism is boosted and you can burn even more calories."

She proposes, "Do you want to talk more body composition for a second?"

Sure, sure, why not. I don't know about the others in this group, but I'm thinking of my own muscles. Could they really go to work for me even when I'm sitting still at the computer? Should I take advantage of the new gym opening up on Route 23 in Cedar Grove near my home in New Jersey which will be offering weight training? To wear a size 10 and not watch calories religiously is most women's dream come true. "Body composition is really so important," Tamara explains, "because you'll get away from the preoccupation with your weight versus height, and get off the scale. Think about it: Thin doesn't necessarily mean healthy. Even if you are successful in dieting yourself down to some god-awfully small size, you could be in terrible shape. Some of those same women who fall into acceptable height/weight categories on paper are unhealthy. Look at the epidemic of anorexia and bulimia among young women."

Tamara outlines two big concepts to remember when thinking about your body composition: lean body mass and body fat. She passes out handouts to stow in the glossy folders that were distributed to everyone at the first session. These packets grow thicker as the weeks go by.

Lean body mass consists of your muscles, bones, nervous tissue, blood, skin, organs, and all that good stuff. All body fat is not bad. Fat's primary role is to store energy for later use. However, there are two kinds of body fat: essential and storage. The essential fat is the amount necessary for maintaining your life and your reproductive functions. It insulates your nerves and protects vital organs, and if you eliminate all of it, you die. Storage fat is the fat contained in pads beneath your skin and surrounding your organs. Too much storage fat equals obesity.

If I've made this evening session sound like a lecture, please forgive me. It wasn't. Discussion about fat, muscle, and exercise in scientific terms continues until nearly 9:00, but it is not a typical classroom setting emotionally. "Sharing and caring," Tamara keeps insisting, "that's what we are here for. We need this place to come to so we can get support for the rest of the week." In fact, Anne, who has missed several recent gatherings because of a new work schedule, laughs about her elderly mother's Fat Chat suspicions.

"After the last session I attended, my mother was so nosy," she explained. "'What is it that you girls do there?' she asked me when I arrived home, as usual, all smiley and happy. 'You are always so happy after Fat Chat. Are you sure you're just talkin'?'"

Linda chimes in, "I told my doctor I was going to Fat Chat, and I think it scared him. I'm a Type II diabetic, and I used to be so worried about my weight. Since I've been exercising and relaxing about what I eat, I've been able to control the diabetes, and I don't have to take the pills the way my mother does or give myself the shots the way my grandfather did. I've lost twenty-five pounds since I met Tamara.

That's about two pounds a month. At the doctor's office, I stepped onto the scale and he said, 'Congratulations,' but I hardly even realized it was happening. When I told him I had learned that it was OK to be me, to love myself just the way I was, and that I was reading labels and moving my body a little bit more every day, he answered, 'Well in that case, Fat Chat is OK.' I can even put a little sugar on my cereal if I want it now."

Peggy says, "I must say that I still hop onto the scale too much. Sometimes when I try to think of what I really want out of all this, I realize that my dream is not to lose weight so much but to get rid of my obsession. I am obsessed with food, which leads to my compulsion to eat. Then I feel guilty, and I want instant results. I push myself hard to walk, go to water aerobics, sign up for the gym, and do more, more, more . . . too much, in fact. Then, I give up and stop everything. It's the obsession that I've got to get rid of. All the women I know are obsessed with how to eat, how to exercise, what society says to look like. EEEEeeeeoooo. Next week I turn forty, and I didn't want to be fat and forty. Yet, here I am."

> *If you have been a yo-yo dieter, it takes time for your injured metabolism to heal and get raised back up to normal. This can take you from 8 to 14 months of normal eating. But, if you just keep eating normally, your metabolism will recover . . . .*
>
> VIKKI HANSEN AND SHAWN GOODMAN,
> *The Seven Secrets of Slim People*

Tamara's Journey . . . in Her Own Words

A Chinese Buffet Restaurant on Washington Road in Augusta:

I went to Weight Watchers once a week after that first session I attended with my neighbor in 1992. That was my beginning. Honestly, seriously, it was the start of my no-turning-back journey. I stood in line for the ritual weigh-in and followed the plan faithfully. In three months, I lost thirty-two pounds. I know what you are thinking here: losing those pounds must have felt great. Sure, it did, but as the group leader would oooohhh and ahhhh when I was on the scale being weighed, I hated it. I can remember thinking, "Why am I letting these three numbers rule my life?" I would want to scream, "There has to be a better way!!!"

You are straitjacketed and without power to control your own life when you give the rights to your body over to someone else. Weight Watchers was a fabulous start for me as well as for millions of others. Yet, I kept thinking (and you should too): "Is this something I can do for the rest of my life and enjoy it? I don't even *like* salad." I was forcing myself every step of the way. I wasn't gaining the new skills I needed to continue on my own journey. I wasn't gaining enough information about body composition or exercise. I had started walking with my ex-husband, but I hadn't reached a real turning point yet. What was missing was the voice inside my own head that had to be saying, "Hey, I'm in control here. I have the power. Nobody else."

Isn't it so true? Turning points are tricky. It is absolutely easier not to take responsibility for your own health. We all want to be struck by that proverbial bolt of enlightenment. Or, maybe we need to hit rock bottom. Or maybe somebody we love has to die first.

Inertia . . . lack of skill 1: a property of matter by which it remains at rest or in uniform motion in the same straight line unless acted upon by some external force 2: indisposition to motion, exertion, or change

WEBSTER'S DICTIONARY

Perhaps my turning point will motivate others to look hard for their own. Mine came when the army transferred my ex-husband to Frankfurt, Germany. Deep down, I knew enough was enough, and I had been at rock bottom after my mother's funeral. In Germany, however, it was panic that pushed me to turn my life around forever. Yes, I said panic. This was the spring of 1992, and there were a lot of reasons I might have been panicky. I was leaving the United States, my family, and my friends and would be eight thousand miles away. My asthma was acting up like crazy, and I could hardly breathe. I couldn't speak German. Telephoning wasn't as cheap as it is now, so I would not be speaking with loved ones very often. All these were causes for panic, but what really, deep, deep, deep, deep down made me panic was that I thought I might not be able to maintain my weight loss without Weight Watchers.

I called their toll-free number before we departed to obtain listings of European groups and discovered that there was a Weight Watchers right in Frankfurt. Whewww. Good thing, I thought. When we arrived, I learned that it had closed. I got really scared. I still weighed more than 200 pounds, and you must know how that feels. I just didn't want to creep back up. The nearest group met at least an hour's drive away from the base, and there was no way I could get there. "Oh my God," I can remember thinking, "I'm sabotaged!" This was my mind-set: negative, dependent, powerless.

What happened after that was simply amazing. In the immediate weeks and then months after we arrived in Germany, my weight stayed the same. I didn't lose any more, but I didn't gain any pounds, either. Can you believe this? I had never experienced anything like it before. Was there something in the European water? Or was there something different about me?

It *was* me. I was moving. I wasn't suffering. I wasn't starving. I was enjoying myself. I was getting out and about because I didn't have a car. In Germany, I had to walk more than I ever did in South Carolina. I recall thinking, "Jeez, this really isn't so hard; I can do this." Little by little, in small daily changes, I altered my daily life. Take butter, for example. We had always been a family that loved butter. Did I used to have a little bread with my butter?!!! Gawwd, yes. What I began to learn was that it was certainly OK to have butter, but not in the extreme quantities I had been eating back home. Whole milk was another point of change. I began buying the 2-percent-fat kind. I still don't buy the skim. I was experimenting and looking for nutritious ways to alter my family's eating patterns. I took a slow, positive, and healthy approach.

After a few more months, the pounds started to drop off dramatically. My metabolism must have shifted. I loved what I was doing in my life. I was eating what I wanted and not what someone else told me to eat. I wasn't overeating, and because I was moving my body, I was able to burn calories and have so much more energy. Our three-bedroom apartment on base was on the third floor, so I had to climb stairs all the time. I walked to the PX to buy essentials. I lugged groceries in a little metal cart, back and forth, up and down. I lifted kids into and out of strollers, and my life was full of movement.

Had I been in Georgia, South Carolina, or Minnesota, I'd have been in the car, still stuck in the notion that exercise is an ugly word or something to be scheduled into my day. Do you know that there are people in my neighborhood who use their cars to get to the mailbox at the end of their driveways? I was in Germany and taking very simple steps.

My child-care load had lightened, which also helped. I had responsibility for only four children because my oldest son had decided to stay with his father, my first husband, back in Minnesota. I wasn't a home-day-care provider, so I had more time for myself. Honestly, as I began to enjoy moving and stopped looking for quick fixes to my fat, I could see that one of the keys to any long-lasting approach to health had to be, "Move it to lose it!"

I've spent a lot of time reading and researching obesity in the years since then, and one of the fascinating areas of clinical study today is the impact your brain has on your body. Because the brain works a bit like a computer, whenever you add new programs for new activities, you begin to change the way it works. Nerve cells are interconnected and forming new connections all the time. Think of your brain as a muscle. When you work it, stretching to learn new facts or new movements, you can transform the chemistry. That's why a brisk walk, a workout, or any kind of exercise can clear your head.

New research in obesity is leading us toward drugs that can begin the miracle of good health right inside your brain. Scientists at the Salk Institute for Biological Studies recently discovered that physical and mental exercise can promote the growth of new brain cells and boost the power of the ones you already have.

The researchers were surprised by their findings but I'm not. I'm living proof. An ancient Buddhist text decrees that all we are is the sum of all we have thought. I began thinking positive in Germany, and the result was simply miraculous. "Love self" became another important principle for me.

It's true that most achievements are the result of many small steps. But if you're stuck on the first step, there's nothing wrong with jumping to the middle.

KATE WHITE, EDITOR OF
COSMOPOLITAN MAGAZINE

I hadn't ridden a bike for more than twenty years, but we purchased a big, black mountain bicycle in Germany so I could get around.

It was cheap transportation, and I used it as a vehicle. I bought those baskets for the sides so I could carry more groceries, and I had a big basket up front as well as the baby carrier on the back. I can remember the first time I climbed on. My muscles hadn't been worked in quite that way for years and years. The seat was wide, and the whole bike was big, built for someone like me. I would hurt and get exhausted, but then I'd get better. I still weighed close to 200 pounds, so I was a big gal wearing about a size 20. My mind was in the right place, and I gave up caring about what I looked like on the bike. You know, I really loved that bike. I'd bring it into the apartment every night because I didn't want to leave it outside. Picture this, if you can, so you can get up on your own bike or march into that exercise class or gym. If I can do it, so can you.

In Europe, there are wonderful bakeries on almost every corner in a town, and one of the most positive images I want to leave you with here is this: me, on my bike, riding to the bakery for fresh bread and sweet rolls.

To find a career to which you are adapted by nature, and then to work hard at it, is about as near to a formula for success and happiness as the world provides. One of the fortunate aspects of this formula is that, granted the right career has been found, the hard work takes care of itself. Then hard work is not hard work at all.

MARK SULLIVAN, *THE FORBES SCRAPBOOK OF THOUGHTS ON THE BUSINESS OF LIFE*

4

To Lose 100 Pounds . . .

"I Focused on My Positive Points"

The Person

Finding out what is important is a fundamental factor in all planning. Often, though, we're too distracted by crisis, by the desire not to think but to do, by the rush and tumble of our everyday lives, to figure out what "important" is.

STEPHAN RECHTSCHAFFEN, M.D., *TIME SHIFTING*

Stuck in Traffic in New York City:

Tamara and I are sitting in my car on Eleventh Avenue inching our way down to the Lincoln Tunnel so we can head back out to my house in New Jersey. It's 3:30 on a Friday afternoon, and everyone else in Manhattan seems to have been struck with the same idea to escape the city early. We have lost the battle to beat the rush-hour traffic, and the streets are packed. Cars are not moving. I surmise that there must be some kind of police action or accident up ahead. I'm not happy, and

I have no energy to spare. We've been on our feet from early in the morning, speaking to people about her Fat Chat program. My mind is numb, and all I want is a nap.

Not Tamara. She is remarkably energized and laughing as she retraces our steps through the last appointment. "Did you see how desperately skinny those three young women were?" she asks me, referring to the executives we had met earlier in an eighth-floor conference room in Times Square. "They all looked as if they had anorexia. And dressed all in black, too! Why do so many professional women in New York City wear all black?"

"Makes them look skinnier?" I suggest. "Takes the guesswork out of getting dressed early in the morning," I add, yawning.

The physical contrast between Tamara—outfitted today in a navy blue and white polka-dot suit, with blonde curly hair, high heels, and stockings—and everyone else who has crossed our path that day is rather astounding. I'm wearing black, too. I look over at her and can see that black is not her color. She's just too happy. It's not that I'm unhappy. I suppose I buy and wear black because I'm trying to fit in, while Tamara always wants to stand out. Could I picture her choosing a black suit from the rack at Daffy Dan's Clothing Bargains for Millionaires where we browsed earlier today? Not really. Her favorite colors, she says, are purple, red, and yellow: "I think those colors are happy and make you feel better than plain black and navy." I wore plain navy yesterday.

"People do stop and stare at me on the street now, don't they?" she asks. Yes, they do. Bemused, she says, "It wasn't that long ago that I had doors slam in my face. Jeez, it wasn't as if the person in front of me couldn't see me coming. I was as big as a house. Now things have changed. Some people might think I've got a perfect body now. I don't. I hate that expression—*perfect body!*—don't you? Yecch. I have an average body just like you and all the other women I meet. I know, I know: compared with where I was eight years ago, there is a big difference. I'm exercising and eating a balanced diet, and I feel strong and confident enough to be telling others how to get healthy, but that doesn't mean I'm a size 4, 6, or 8. Weren't those women thin?" she says again.

If you give, you will receive, perhaps not from the same source and not in the same way, but giving is always returned. That is an

unwritten law. If you put out negatives, you get negatives back.
Conversely, if you put out positives, only positives will return.

ARLENE DAHL, *BEYOND BEAUTY*

"Why is it that society has this impossible insistence on there being some kind of perfect body? The definition of what constitutes beauty or even an acceptable body seems to become more inaccessible every year. Constantly bombarded by perfect body images on TV, in movies, on magazine covers, and everywhere we look, we can't see that these high-fashion images have been airbrushed to create a supernatural person. Those women whose shapes we worship have had breast implants, liposuction, and cosmetic surgery. Professional makeup artists spend hours getting them ready for on-camera appearances. We look down at our real thighs and wish them away. We dream irrationally of having those stick legs depicted in the sale catalogs that land in our mail piles," she says, going a mile a minute. The car has been between Forty-Seventh and Forty-Sixth Streets for at least twenty minutes. We are going nowhere.

"Do you know that experts estimate that consumers are bombarded with more than two thousand advertising images every single day?" she asks.

"No, I didn't know that."

As I've seen all day long in presentations, Tamara loves to use statistics in her sales pitch. She pulls these numbers out of her brain easily and often. I'm impressed.

- Six out of every ten people are physically inactive and exercise very seldom.
- In 1995, an estimated 300,000 people died from diseases directly related to obesity.
- Fifty-eight million Americans are considered obese.
- The diet industry is huge. It's a $45 billion-a-year business.
- There are about 80 million people dieting all the time.
- Of those dieters, 95 percent gain back every pound they have lost within five years.
- There is no one like me. I've had babies. I've lost 100 pounds and kept that weight off.

Yes, she is a statistic: one of a kind. Tamara will stand up dramatically and, with her hands on her hips, raise her voice pleasantly but insistently and describe herself as the average American woman. "You must listen to me," she says. "I represent women all across the United States. *Me*. This is what fit looks like. This is what health looks like. This is what weight loss and maintenance are all about.

"I insist on talking about fat very frankly," she continues. "My whole program is me chatting with you about *fat*, sharing my secrets of success and caring about others so very much. I don't want to duck the issue of fat. I know what it feels like. Say it out loud. *Fat*. I want people to say it so they can start doing something about it.

"All bodies have good and bad points. Measuring yourself against an unrealistic standard of beauty beamed into your life over and over again is a losing battle. These images set the average woman up to fail. Unless you are genetically destined to be 5'10" and 110 pounds with those Barbie doll legs, you can't win. The average height and weight of an American woman is 5'4" and 142 pounds. The average height and weight of a model is that incredible, unreachable 5'10" and 110 pounds. Her measurements are 33"–23"–33". She's probably starving herself to stay there and not very happy. Those rail-thin women comprise only 2 percent of the population."

Tamara has hips as wide as her strong shoulders. A powerful figure, she is soft and womanly, too. "Most women put on weight easily, and for many, it goes straight to the midsection or hips. We are supposed to be curvy," she says.

The culture, she says, is unhealthy. "American women are feeling worse and worse about their average, normal bodies. Our society has evolved into a world that worships and approves an unnatural view of beauty. That perfect-body standard is just short of starvation for most women. And believe me, young women are starving themselves sick. All the weight loss in the world won't help you if you don't love yourself for who you are," she says. "There is no perfect body despite society's insistence to the contrary. We all have to stop trying to achieve the unattainable because it is making us sicker and sicker. You wreak havoc on your metabolism when you starve and binge, starve and binge, lose and gain, gain and lose."

No one can make you feel inferior without your consent.

ELEANOR ROOSEVELT

We reach the Lincoln Tunnel entrance finally, and she relaxes a little. "I'm hungry," she says. "Can we stop at Dunkin' Donuts on the way home?"

"You are amazing," I say.

The Program

Our images of womanhood are almost synonymous with thinness. If we are thin, we shall feel healthier, lighter, and less restricted. Our sex lives will be easier and more satisfying. We shall have more energy and vigor. We shall be able to buy nice clothes and decorate our bodies, winning approval from our lovers, families, and friends. We shall be the woman in the advertisements who lives the good life; we shall be able to project a variety of images—athletic, sexy, or elegant. We shall set a good example to our children. No doctors will ever again yell at us to take off the excess weight. We shall be beautiful. We shall never have to be ashamed about our bodies, at the beach, in a store trying to buy clothes, or in a tightly packed automobile. . . ."

SUSIE ORBACH, *FAT IS A FEMINIST ISSUE*

Powerhouse Gym in the Washington Road Shopping Center:

It's crowded on a Monday evening. The large, L-shaped, gray-carpeted, mirror-lined main room is brightly lit. Ooooo . . . the space makes a newcomer like me want to shrink back in fear . . . fear of looking stupid or actually falling off one of these machines.

Six rows of exercise machines are almost all in use by men and a trickle of thin women who apparently know what they are doing, working muscles they understand perfectly. A free-weight area, populated by big guys who are lifting bars, pumping biceps, and who knows what else, is located to the right and in the rear of the gym. That space, over there, is definitely an all-male preserve, my mind clicks adamantly.

Are we in the right place? Fat Chat here? In a gym called Power-house? Whoooaaa, as Tamara would say; these images are at odds with each other. I walk and play a little tennis in my local public park on weekday mornings when I am at home in New Jersey, so I'm no stranger to exercise. But still, this place is kind of scary at first glance.

"Relax," she says. "This will be fun."

Wearing a T-shirt that surely sums up her message: Exercise Is Ter-minal Wellness, she is right at home amid the activity. Friends call out to her. The manager hollers hello. I'd say that she is the fearless leader every woman needs when entering such a predominantly male testos-terone zone. Her posture speaks volumes about her confidence. It rubs off. My fear of looking like a fool disappears. Then, she spots two of her Fat Chat gals at work. Amy and Marilyn are far from skinny, and yet both are at home here, getting stronger, using the buddy system as they venture into what may have once felt like forbidden territory. Standing near an eight-foot-high chrome and steel Modular Power Assist Dip machine, Amy tells me, "I feel so good about what I can do now. I am much stronger than I've been in years, and I've lost inches. Want to try this one?" I'm relieved that not everyone in the gym tonight is already in shape.

Later, we chat. This is the fourth week of the formal program being offered here at Powerhouse Gym, and tonight's topic is self-acceptance. "We've been taking some simple steps along the way here, every day," Tamara explains to me. "When I was 250 pounds, I had no place to go, no understanding of where to begin except taking away calories. That was so wrong. The first week, we talked about taking ourselves out of denial, and then we spent some time on self-awareness, and last week, the group spent time setting goals."

In Fat Chat, Tamara teaches that a goal is a predetermined idea directed toward a desired result. You take home a handout so you can spend time on your own defining your goals. Be careful. Your goal is not a picture of what you want to do, to be, to get, or to achieve. It is a target. Goals start in your heart. To have goals that are really mean-ingful, you need to be in touch with what matters to you and what you want. It is extremely important that you give a lot of thought to exactly what you want to do.

"Sometimes, there are things in our lives that can block us from achieving what we want or what we want to be," Tamara says. "Past learning and experiences keep all of us from moving ahead. Sometimes we set the wrong goals. Such goals might be unrealistic or unachievable. Other times, we let other people set our goals." She notes that not being able to focus on your positive points can keep you from progressing.

> *Don't allow self-pity. The moment this emotion strikes, do something nice for someone less fortunate than you.*
>
> H. JACKSON BROWN JR., *LIFE'S LITTLE INSTRUCTION BOOK*

"We've got goal fever tonight," Tamara says. "Having goals can be very exciting and motivating. A goal isn't ever going to be a burden. The opposite is true. There are two kinds of goals I recommend setting," Tamara explains. Last week, the assignment was to look for short-term as well as long-term goals. "Short-term goals keep you encouraged, self-motivated, and on target. Long-term goals give your life meaning and direction."

To set goals on your own, keep Tamara's guidelines in mind:

- Conceivable—Anything that can be imagined is possible. You must be able to picture it clearly in your mind.
- Believable—You must be able to imagine yourself achieving it, having it, or doing it.
- Specific—Your goals must say exactly what you want to do. They can't be general.
- Achievable—They must fit your abilities, strengths, present condition, level of motivation, and time.
- Measurable—They must be stated so that they can be measured in both quantity and time. They must say how much you're going to do, when you will start working, and when you will have them accomplished.
- Goals are much more likely to be met if they are committed to paper.

"Did you write yours down?" Tamara asks.

Every woman has a weight that is ideal for her, as opposed to an ideal weight. This is the weight at which you feel the most

*comfortable, have the most energy, can stay well, and feel good
about how you look. . . . Instead of weighing yourself, let your
favorite clothes tell how you are doing.*

SARAH BAN BREATHNACH,
SIMPLE ABUNDANCE

"When I first started working with Amy and Marilyn," Tamara
recalls, "they could hardly lift five-pound dumbbells in an overhead
press. In a bench press, lying flat on their backs with the bar at forty-
five pounds, they were both wobbling crazily after only one repetition
and with my help. Now they are both up to ten pounds with free
weights and can do five or six repetitions easily. When benching, they'll
do sixty pounds on their own, and I'm not even assisting anymore. Doctors say that women should be able to bench one time their own body
weight. There is no physical or skeletal reason why we can't."

Marilyn describes a side effect of her recent efforts: "I used to get
out of breath running up and down the steps in my house after the dog.
I would be huffing and puffing and have to go slow. I couldn't keep up
with the dog. I work from home, and now I can chase after that dog
upstairs or downstairs with no problem. I feel really, really good about
this." To chase the dog without getting winded! How's that for a goal?

"I tell people over and over again that you may not be able to see
or gauge specific gains in strength until you do some specific activity
or chore that once tired you out. Waxing floors or vacuuming requires
a lot of upper-arm strength," Tamara says. Getting strong is going to
help in every area of life, according to Tamara's mantra. So, forget the
scale, focus on good health, and remember the three basic principles:
Love self. Think health. Move it to lose it. She emphasizes, "When I
was a big woman, I could hardly lift my legs. The pressure on my knees
and lower back was tremendous. It happens with lots of fat people."

"Hey, did Tamara tell you her trick with the scale?" someone asks,
turning to me. She has. During the sixteen-week course, originally
designed for Aiken Regional Medical Centers, participants are measured
and weighed at least twice, but the goal is never to focus on the numbers alone. For this reason, you climb onto the scale backward for the
first weigh-in so you can't look down and be pulled down emotionally by the weight of those numbers. Tamara records the actual amount,
and a few weeks later, after a second weigh-in, also "blind," the good
news can sound really good.

"I know it sounds crazy, but this simple little thing puts the emphasis on the positive," she explains. "No one has to see those three numbers. All they need to see is success. I can say, 'Wow, you've lost two, three, four, or five pounds,' instead of announcing the figure in full. I remember when I first started to go to Weight Watchers and I'd look at 253, 251, 247 on the scale: how could that get me excited? The group leader might say, 'Ooooo Tamara, look where you are?' But all I could focus on was how far I had to go. How could that possibly make me feel good? What I've learned is that your attitude is almost everything."

In sessions like number four tonight, women learn that they tell the world how awful they may feel about their bodies without ever saying a word out loud. Tamara illustrates: "Do you walk with shoulders hunched? Head down? Chin to chest? Does your stature say, 'I don't like my body very much. It's not perfect.' My God, girl, give up that thinking!

"Call me Sergeant Hill," she says. "I don't care."

Quick. Pull those shoulders back. Hold your head high. Put your chin up. A confident stature can speak louder than your size. Honestly, as our fearless leader proves, good posture and knowing how to accentuate your body's positive points can make a profound difference.

Even when she was 200-plus pounds, daytime television talk show host Ricki Lake would walk into a room, and all heads would turn. She was so positive. So stunning.

Tamara's Journey . . . in Her Own Words

At the La Quinta Inn in Augusta:

In years past, medicine ignored our unique individuality. Our bodies were treated like machinery, needing repairs only after breaking down. It was like going to the body shop to fix your car, as though hearts were like engines.

REED MOSKOWITZ, M.D.,
YOUR HEALING MIND

I got a part-time job stocking shelves and working as a cashier in the commissary when I was in Germany in 1992. I could ride my big, black bike to and from work, and my hours were flexible enough so that my ex-husband could be home taking care of the kids. Out, about, and moving, I've always been a talker, but now I was talking to other adults. It was exhilarating. You should try it. What I discovered as I began to focus on myself, my positive points, and what I really liked to do was that I stopped being as hungry for food.

During that year of experimenting, I progressed from a woman who fed herself for emotional reasons to someone who ate—most of the time—to sustain life. Not that I don't enjoy food. I still love to eat, but food ceased to be the center of my life. Eating was something I did when I was hungry and not just because it happened to be mealtime. I also learned to recognize those hunger signals.

Some people say that fat people hide in their large sizes. I'm not sure this is true, but I will say that I had grown comfortable with the idea of being fat. There was a certainty about it. It was me. Of course, you and I both know that any kind of change is fearful. How would people perceive me if I were thinner? Would I still be the same person? Losing weight was an unknown. Perhaps it was safer to stay fat, but I also knew that I couldn't afford to end up like my mother. Who would take care of my children?

With me, I was simply blind to my situation, as well. I was a big woman who had thought she was much smaller. Fat can protect you. It's a very useful device because when you are fat, people don't always take you as seriously as they should, so you just don't try. As I lost weight, my life changed dramatically. No, it wasn't as scary as you might think. Yes, it was hard but not as painfully difficult as you may be imagining. My journey was and still is quite wonderful.

Diets provide people with feelings of failure, fustration and discouragement. Indeed, unrealistic, impractical diet plans are prescriptions for failure.

LYNN J. BENNION, M.D., EDWIN L.
BIERMAN, M.D., AND JAMES M. FERGUSON,
M.D., *STRAIGHT TALK ABOUT WEIGHT CONTROL*

There was a point late in the fall of 1992 when I was really relying on my instincts and learning more about myself every day. Another gal on base with me who was much younger and big, too, noticed that I was losing weight and became curious. Though she was interested in what I was doing, she was iffy about making a commitment for her own health. As I've said before, you are either ready or not. I can help you along the way. My story can inspire you because if I can do it, then so can others. I can even lift you up a little, but I can't go deep inside you to make you do something for yourself. Your motivation has to come from within yourself.

My friend in Germany didn't want to change, and I couldn't empower her. To be honest, I don't think she had been fat long enough. In her early twenties and the mother of only one little child, she hadn't reached that gut-wrenching despair I knew so well. In high school, she had been thin. She didn't know the agony I had lived through at my mother's funeral. I would encourage her to walk with me, but that's about as far as she went.

Meanwhile, my clothes were getting looser. Every time I dropped down a size, I'd treat myself to an item of clothing: a pair of new jeans, a shirt, just something new. You don't have to spend a lot of money, but building rewards into your progress is important. Even time away from a busy schedule may be reward enough to make you smile. Rent a movie. Read a book. I celebrated my successes, and you should, too.

What did I do with my fat clothes? I just couldn't keep them in my closet because I had decided that I'd never go back, and I didn't want to leave the clothes there staring at me. There was no turning back, no looking back, and the clothes might tempt me with an option I didn't want around. So, I gave them to my fat friend. Maybe once a month, after I had lost another ten, fifteen, twenty pounds, I'd drop by her home with a bag of clothes. The feeling was exhilarating for me, and she was happy to have them. I was like a kid with a new bike, on my own bike when I'd take those things to her. Thank goodness, she never made me feel uncomfortable or tried to sabotage my efforts. She just wasn't in the same place mentally that I had found in Germany. She had to search harder or suffer longer before reaching her turning point.

Anyway, after stopping to see her and leaving my "goodie" bag, I'd go on over to the PX, looking excited. Sometimes, people would say, "Well, look at you. You're losing weight. What are you doing?"

I guess it was hard not to notice the changes in me. Even my ex-husband's soldier friends could comment, "Your wife is looking good." This definitely fed my soul, though it proved to be the beginning of the end of my marriage. I also knew that while compliments were great and heartfelt, losing the weight was for me and no one else. Don't expect compliments in your own journey.

> *Girls are socialized to look to the world for praise and rewards,*
> *and this keeps them other-oriented and reactive. . . . Look*
> *within yourself for validation.*
>
> MARY PIPHER, PH.D., *REVIVING OPHELIA*

One of the women who wrote to me last year has a story that illustrates perfectly well how expecting approval and compliments can backfire. She lost 100 pounds through Weight Watchers and was so excited about her success that she shared her enthusiasm with her father, who is obese. Though she had anticipated his approval, all she got were his nasty comments that she would eventually gain it all back, accompanied by his prediction that she'd always have problems with excess weight. His negative pronouncements were so awful. Now she has put the pounds back on, and every time she thinks about getting healthy again, she remembers her father's words dooming her to failure, so she gives up. The voice inside her head is not her own but her dad's.

What I learned in my journey is that I had to forget the compliments as well as the snide remarks from naysayers. I held my head up high. When I stopped concentrating on looking good for others to see the "outside me" and started putting all my efforts into wellness and the "inside me," I began to feel better emotionally as well as physically.

This power to lose weight was in me. I saw those pounds go off, and I could still have German strudel at the corner bakery.

5

To Lose 100 Pounds . . .

"I Learned There Is Nothing Evil About Food"

The Person

The Chinese Buffet Restaurant at Noon:

Buffets are big in the South. Twice in September, Tamara and I have stood before this smorgasbord of selections with stomachs growling. There's nothing like real hunger at this Chinese all-you-can-eat buffet. I wonder if the guy behind the steam table can actually hear the pops and gurgles of my digestive system clamoring for comfort. I can't decide what should fill my plate. "Look at those fried pork dumplings!" Chicken wings, BBQ spareribs, cold noodles with sesame sauce, chicken with cashew nuts, beef with snow pea pods, shrimp in lobster sauce, broccoli in garlic sauce, rice and more fried rice . . .

We coo, oooh, and chatter back and forth to each other cruising along the line of scrumptious offerings with our trays. There is only one other table of patrons already seated, and the hostess recognizes us from earlier in the week. It's quiet here, and I've brought my tape recorder so we can continue our chat session begun earlier in my hotel room.

"I think I'm going to have some of the tempura. I love the deep fried shrimp. What do you think?"

"Sounds great."

A little voice inside my head starts whispering no-no's. "This sauce has got to be full of fat," I say.

"I don't care," Tamara replies. "I'm going to put some on my rice."

Later, back at work, our talk turns to the topic of food and how women are caught in a web of guilt, gain, lose, guilt, and so on and so forth. "Yadda, yadda, yadda," as Tamara says. Recalling our earlier conversation at the buffet, Tamara says, "Can't you see what was going on? Though you were legitimately hungry, standing before wholesome, interesting, nutritious food, you let guilt get in the way of your satisfaction before you had even taken a single bite. Girl, all of us have been so brainwashed for so many years that we carry around a load of angst whenever we think of or look at food. If we feel this way—and neither of us is overweight now—then imagine the guilt of the person who is obese. It's unreasonable. It's obscene. There's nothing evil about food. Oh Lord, this is the kind of mentality that keeps people fat."

> *Getting in touch with your feelings may seem like a Herculean task if you've spent much of your life trying to avoid them, but it can be done.*
>
> SARAH, DUCHESS OF YORK, IN *DIETING WITH THE DUCHESS*

Tamara advocates a guilt-free approach. "The world looks at a fat person and thinks, 'This is a bad person, a lazy person. You must want to be fat. You deserve to be fat.' You are not a bad or lazy person because you are fat," she insists. "You may not even be overeating at all but could be stuck in a daily pattern that has become dangerous to your mental and physical health. You don't choose to be fat, and you shouldn't feel guilty.

"The women in my Fat Chat sessions start to dig beneath the surface of their lives to find out where they are getting stuck or off track in terms of health. I have everyone fill out a questionnaire that gets them to thinking. Small steps make a big difference. Little meals. No starvation. Small moves. All day long. You don't need to become overzealous. I help them look for a turning point—a catalyst that will change their lives."

She emphasizes, "There is no immediate gratification in this game, though the media promise a quick fix constantly. I'm not some person on a Slim Fast commercial who lost 50 pounds and says, 'Here, drink this.' Let's go talk to that individual in two years and see just how healthy he or she still is."

Tamara says, "I'm an expert because I was 100 pounds heavier and so unhealthy. I didn't love myself. I didn't take care of myself. I didn't think I deserved to take care of myself. When I started losing weight and experiencing exercise, I found myself. I've kept that weight off for more than six years, and to me, that makes an expert! I've been experted!" she says with a laugh. "And I didn't lose that weight by dieting!"

> *We may want money, we may want recognition, we may want sex, and we may want to be thinner. But what we really want is to be happy.*
>
> COLLEEN DUNN BATES, "IS EVERY-
> BODY HAPPY?" *WEIGHT WATCHERS*
> MAGAZINE

Her communication skills, she reveals, go way back. "I was always very approachable," Tamara confides. "Here's a true and funny little story about myself that my mother told me before she passed away. When I was a tiny, little snow-white blonde girl, we lived on a corner lot in Granite Falls, Minnesota. I was the baby; my siblings were all older. My mother would find me out at the end of our yard trying to stop strangers on the street to listen to me speak. One day, someone came to the door and asked my mother just how old I was. When she told them I was only three, the person couldn't believe that I was able to speak so eloquently. I've just always had the gift of gab."

The Program

> *People who have a goal or who are engaged in a cause, crusade, hobby or relationship that deeply matters to them are healthier,*

happier, more resilient, joyful and alive. Going for our dreams means going with our natural flow, unleashing the energy, talents, abilities, vision and initiatives within us.

JACKI NINK PFLUG, *MILES TO GO*
BEFORE I SLEEP

Betty's Kitchen in Aiken, South Carolina:

Betty is one of Tamara's most loyal exercise-class participants. Retired and slim, Betty jokes that what she really wants Tamara to give her are rock-hard abs, buns of steel, and one of those stomachs that you can bounce a quarter off. What she is getting from Tamara after a year's worth of evening classes is energy, stamina, and upper-body strength. "She used to enjoy raking, weeding, and planting," Tamara explained, "but it would hurt or she'd run out of steam before finishing a project. I think people do less and less when they develop sore muscles, and then, compounded with age, they start to lose so much muscle and bone mass. For women in Betty's age range, osteoporosis can be a real threat, but it's never too late to combine aerobics with strength training, which is exactly what I do in my classes."

After class one Thursday evening, Betty invites the crowd of Fat Chat crew mixed with aerobics students to share a potluck supper at her house. Still in sweaty gear, we form a caravan of cars and pull into a lovely wooded suburban area. Sheri, Becky, Nancy, Amy, Christa, Wanda, and I chat with Tamara around a dining table. Someone mentions that the media have been calling Monica Lewinsky fat. "Monica Lewinsky is not fat. She is average," Tamara insists. "In Europe, magazines are clamoring for her to model. Just because she has boobs and hips, here in America she's called fat, fat, fat and it's terribly unfair."

We are eating. We are eating. With full plates around a long table, we tease Tamara about what she might look like in real clothes versus the exercise outfits in which she lives. We also cajole her about her eating habits because she is definitely not someone who tortures herself calorically. "Food is not your enemy," she protests. "Nor is it the answer to your problems. In fact, it's that kind of thinking that can get us all in trouble. You've got to eat for your health as well as for enjoyment," she says, and it's clear she practices what she preaches.

Snacking is great. More people should be encouraged to grab a bite instead of waiting until the next meal. A snack can keep you from binging when you get too hungry. And snacking is a good way to pay more attention to what your body is telling you—to recognize when you're hungry and to eat only as much as you need to satisfy yourself.

JOHN LA PUMA, ALEXIAN BROTHERS
MEDICAL CENTER, CHICAGO

"There is no such thing as a forbidden food," Tamara maintains. "You've all seen me eat my cashews. I love to snack on nuts when I'm in a pinch and need energy. For sure, cashews are on some experts' 'forbidden' lists, but, nuts are plant foods which means that they are carbohydrates and will provide me with a boost. Sometimes, I'll have peanut butter crackers in my van or something sweet."

The compulsion to rush to the cupboard on a bad day is gone for Tamara, as she explains: "Today, I might say, 'Hey, I feel like having a piece of cake,' so I'll have one, but I'll cut myself a piece and won't have to finish the entire cake and hide the box it came in. Now I know that my body is craving something sweet, and I don't need to deny that craving. There is no more of that restrictive thinking: 'This is what you can eat. This is what you can't eat. Stay away from these forbidden foods. Eat only these foods.'"

The German strudel Tamara ate at the corner bakeries after her bike rides did not make her fat, because she was making healthy choices all day long. "You need to eat your favorite foods, or you'll go crazy," she says. "An excess of foods high in saturated animal fats, when eaten in large quantities over a long period of time when you aren't exercising or moving your body, will contribute to weight gain. The excess will make you fat. But a steak? Will a steak or a piece of cake or strudel make you fat? No way."

She points out, "I forget to eat sometimes—when I'm rushing to class at the hospital or in the middle of a session—and I can feel my energy take a dive." Everyone scoffs at the notion of Tamara's ever being out of energy. "Oh, it happens," she insists, noting, "When I was heavy, I didn't have the kind of energy I have now. It's the exercise and eating right that have given me the energy to go, go, go."

"How do you do it five days a week?" Amy asks. "You pump us up, but where do you go to get pumped up?"

"I don't go anywhere," she replies. "It's in me and is coming from within. I want to give people not only the knowledge but also the inspiration. The average woman is not being motivated by those beautiful people you see at health-club scenes. She needs someone like me, someone who has achieved her goal realistically, slowly, steadily, and without ever considering turning back. I know I've said this before and often, but it's so important: You cannot possibly lose more than two to three pounds of weight in a week and expect to keep it off. You've got to go my way, and I know you can do it because I did."

The fear of certain foods is put into perspective as all of us learn how Tamara put food into perspective in her own life. "Choose a meal plan that will let you eat well," she says. "Make choices about what, when, where, and how much you will eat. For instance, don't deny yourself that Big Mac today. Buy one, but share it with a friend. Give yourself permission to have treats when you want them. You really have got to work at creating a meal plan that makes you happy. If you don't enjoy it, you aren't going to be able to stick with it for the rest of your life. Eating," Tamara repeats, "should not make you feel guilty or unhappy, and guilt about food will only make you have negative feelings about yourself."

According to her premise, feelings of depression, poor self-image, and low self-esteem almost always lead to more overeating which makes you feel worse. Cravings reflect an actual physical need either for a specific nutrient or for food in general. When she began a varied, well-balanced diet and started getting enough food, her own cravings were less powerful than ever before.

"I know you find this hard to believe, but it's true," Tamara tells us. "Emotional cravings for particular foods are not all in your head! They are just as real as the physical kind. We all associate certain foods with comfort and good times, so we crave them when we are under stress. Did you know that high-carbohydrate foods increase your brain's supply of serotonin, a chemical that affects your mood? Ooooh, that's why I reach for a muffin or that glazed doughnut when I'm stressed out."

She offers an example of facing down temptation: "The other night, two of my former Fat Chat ladies were shopping together in the Bi-Lo store and heard an announcement that they almost couldn't resist: the baker had made too many doughnuts, and they were going on sale for half price. They almost rushed over to take advantage of the bargain and gorge themselves immediately. But because they had been coming to class, they knew that eating doughnuts late in the evening was not a good idea. 'We didn't do it, Tamara,' they told me."

In the digestive system, she explains, fat is broken down more slowly than carbohydrates, so after you eat something fatty, you feel fuller longer. Fat also carries flavor and improves texture, which can make foods taste better and be more enjoyable to eat. "You don't have to get rid of all your fatty foods," Tamara says; "just reach for the right kinds."

In formal sessions numbers seven and eight, participants bring in labels from some of their regular grocery-store purchases (see the example in Chapter 9). In the process of learning how to read a nutrition label, definitions fly back and forth, and handouts are provided on fats, carbohydrates, proteins, sugars, cholesterol, fiber, vitamins, and minerals, as well as information about serving sizes, to be slipped into individualized Fat Chat packets. "Everyone is different," says Tamara, "but knowledge about our bodies, nutrition, and exercise is so powerful. Aim low with your fats. Too much in your diet will contribute to heart disease and cancer. Limit and be clear about your choices." She specifically advises, "Go for the kind of oil that will reduce your cholesterol: safflower, corn, soybean, sesame, sunflower, margarine, mayonnaise, olive, canola, and peanut oils."

Yes, some of this feels like work, but her pep keeps these sessions upbeat and fun.

Someone says, "Oh, I remember my first class. I was so embarrassed to be there. Now I know how to read a label. You know, it's the sugar that kicks my butt. Everything has sugar in it . . . pasta sauces and even cereals. Shredded wheat is probably the best. Tamara has provided me with that little voice inside my head. It's there all the time now, even when I'm watching TV. Do you know that I saw Tamara on TV and even tried some of the exercises she was demonstrating. The movements looked pretty easy, and when I saw her program announced in the paper later, I thought, 'This is where I need to be going.'"

Tamara tilts her head and smiles approvingly. It's apparent that the women feel very comfortable in her presence. She states, "I'm living proof that you can eat a normal diet and lose 100 pounds. A piece of paper with a list of foods you must avoid and a limitation of 1,200 calories a day will drive you crazy sooner or later. You and I both know this so well. You simply can't stay motivated by feelings of guilt or deprivation for very long.

"Jeez," she says, "military life wasn't easy. I had all those kids and was in the kitchen preparing meals, cleaning up, making snacks and always getting ready for the next meal. I never went anywhere and I ate because I was unhappy. I'd eat my dessert and then two or three more later. A single serving of that dessert didn't make me fat, and forcing myself to eat grapefruit didn't make me thin. Duh.

"Too many of us want it so easy. We want to do as little as possible. We don't have time. We want to super-size everything. Just think how crazy this is. Everything in excess. For God's sake," she says, growing heated, "you can eat beef, pork, and cake, too. It's all a question of how you buy it, how you prepare it, how often you eat it, and how much of it you eat."

> *The opportunities for enjoyment in your life are limitless. If you feel you are not experiencing enough joy, you have only yourself to blame.*
>
> DAVID E. BRESLER, *QUOTATIONS TO CHEER YOU UP*

Look at some of those restrictive weight-loss regimens, she says. "Saying no, no, no only makes you want to eat those foods even more. In my house now, we make healthier choices. Take the cake I just mentioned: I didn't buy the double-layer chocolate cake. I picked up a vanilla cake with white frosting because the fat content on the labels showed me what I was going to be eating. Sure, the white cake had sugar, but it didn't have all the fat of the chocolate. You don't have to become paranoid about food, but you have to really want to do something for yourself and your health. You can enjoy the benefits of all food groups. You've got to find the foods that work for you. Experiment. I eat anything I want to eat, but just not in excess quantities, and I watch my fats."

Dinner and the dynamics of a casual Fat Chat session have relaxed everyone. "You know," Becky says, "Sheri and I were driving over to the hospital tonight, and I kept saying to her, 'I don't want to do this. How am I going to do this? I'm not going to make it. But now that I'm here, I feel better than I know I would have if I hadn't come."

"That's because of the taco salad I made," someone jokes.

"No, it's because of all of you. I couldn't do this if I didn't have all this support," she says. "Especially you, Tamara."

"I wish Jeri Lyne could have made it tonight," Tamara says, turning to me. "I know I've talked about her. I'm glad she is back in school now, but her schedule means that she can't make these meetings, and I worry about her."

Tamara recaps the story. "I met Jeri Lyne when I spoke at an obesity clinic in Augusta, and she was their star loser. At twenty-eight, she had been up to 326 pounds and a size 30 when she broke both of her legs because of the excess weight. She's a mom with three little ones, ages four, six, and nine now, so she has to get well. She was paying the clinic $125 to $150 a month, where they gave her fen-phen. Her weight loss was so 'successful' that they used her in one of their ads promoting the program, but she had been on a 1,000-to-1,200-calories-a-day diet and couldn't keep on like that. All the clinic was doing for Jeri Lyne was taking away the calories and giving her the pills, which turned out to be dangerous for her health. She learned very little about exercise and focused all her attention on those pounds on the scale, following lists of what she could and couldn't eat.

"When I met her, she had tears in her eyes," Tamara says. "I helped her get off the pills and insisted that she add more calories to her daily diet. Metabolically, with her size, she couldn't exist on those few calories. I remember saying to her, 'Jeri Lyne, can you really take this pill for the rest of your life? Do you think it's feasible or healthy?' I told her the medication may have helped her get started, but it's the exercise and eating right that will give you the feeling of high energy and health that you need to keep right on going.

"Her weight went down to 192 while she was able to keep on coming to Fat Chat sessions, and though she has gone back up a little now that she's in school, she's still on that path to good health. She's got my picture on her dresser mirror so that when she looks at herself, she can look at me at the same time. She claims that I saved her life."

People are the only animals who eat themselves to death.

Tamara's Journey . . . in Her Own Words

On the Phone in My Third-Floor Office:

When I stepped off the plane in New York after a year in Germany, I weighed 150 pounds. Something inside me had changed forever. Honest to God, girl, my mind-set was the biggest, biggest factor in this transformation. It was my attitude and my brainpower, not some diet, that helped me lose those 100 pounds. In the airport, my children ran toward their grandmother, who was there to pick us up. She looked around and started asking, "Where's Mommy? Where's Mommy?" I was right there, wearing a nice suit which had a rather short skirt, and I had on pumps. No one recognized me because I was a size 10 or 12.

Here I was, this lady no one back in the States knew anymore. Because I had been accountable to me and only me, I hadn't shared any of my news with my family or my in-laws. I didn't send photos. I didn't keep them updated. I didn't ask for anyone's approval or invite their disdain. Yes, of course, it's nice to have people congratulate you, and I don't want to sound ungrateful, but if you are true to yourself and what's good for you, then what others think just doesn't matter. Their opinions are unnecessary to your success. You'll do better without them, I suspect.

Isn't it so true? No one else can really understand what you are going through. That's why your plan has to belong to you. You don't want anyone coming back to you, not even me, saying, "Well, exactly how much did you lose? Or yadda, yadda, yadda." What you are doing for your health is for you. I lost those 100 pounds for me and only me.

Right there amid the hustle and bustle of the busy New York City airport while we waited for our luggage, they all looked at me as if I were the product of a miracle. Yes, it was almost as if they believed that my weight loss had come from God. It was so very interesting.

My ex-mother-in-law is a big woman, and so is my ex-husband's youngest sister, who was about thirteen or fourteen years old then. In fact, she may have been more than 300 pounds. They were both in awe of me. We lived with them for several weeks in their home outside New York while we waited for our next military assignment. Their household is not focused entirely on food, but they just don't move a lot, and there are some family and emotional issues that were, and still are, unsettling. Hypersensitive to certain foods, my ex-mother-in-law stays away from sugars and breads, but overall, there is no commitment to good health or eating nutritiously. They would look at me, talk about my weight loss, but think and say, "This is certainly something we can't do."

Unfortunately, my ex-sister-in-law is an emotional eater, and her mom would lock up the food at night. Yes, that's right. Can you imagine? This was a home in which the kitchen had to be locked at night to keep someone out. I haven't seen them since my divorce, but when I look back at this experience, I understand more clearly that the food alone wasn't making her fat. There she was, five foot tall and nearly five foot wide and looking for a miracle. Don't you think that if I had that miracle pill or potion, I'd bottle it to help you as well as all the women like her? Of course I would. If there is a miracle to be had, it's right there in your own head.

> *The Lord gave us two ends—one to sit on and the other to think with. Success depends on which one we use the most.*
>
> ANN LANDERS

Genetic and biological factors can cause obesity, of course, but being fat is so much more complex. I've got lots of obesity genes, but I'm proof that you don't have to follow in your parents' footsteps. The fitness and weight-loss industries try to simplify everything and tell you that if you just take away the calories, you can get thin. You can't win that way. There must be three parts to your plan: Love Self, Think Health, Move It to Lose It. If any one of these is missing, your platform is like a three-legged stool minus one leg. It's not stable, not usable. You'll fall down.

Some women come to me and say that their metabolism is faulty: they can't lose weight because their body's metabolism is too slow. Your metabolism is slow because you aren't moving your body enough and you aren't eating meals throughout the day. I had a gal come up to me in a group session not so long ago who couldn't understand why she was still fat. "Tamara," she said, "I only eat one meal a day about one or two o'clock in the afternoon. I don't understand what's wrong with me."

"Oh my God," I said to her, "there's your miracle answer. You've come to me, the miracle worker, and the miracle cure is right there in your daily lifestyle." I explained, "Your body is staying dormant when you rest at night. You are asleep for six to eight hours and sometimes longer. You haven't had any water. You haven't had any food for fuel. Your system completely slows down at night, bringing your metabolism to a snail's crawl."

Doesn't it make sense to wake it up first thing in the morning? Imagine submerging a person in cold, cold water and forcing all the bodily functions to slow up. The same thing happens to your metabolism. Your heart rate is slowed. Your energy level is way, way down there at the bottom. To bring your metabolism back up, you've got to get up and eat. Eating breakfast will bring your body to life. Feed yourself something, anything—some fruit, a piece of toast. You need little meals all day long, not one in the middle of the day. If you eat only once, you are tricking your metabolism into thinking that you are in a starvation mode where every calorie should be stored as fat.

The next big thing to do in the morning is to move. Go up and down your stairs. Do some housework. Finish those dishes from the night before. Throw in a load of laundry. Twist and shout. Park your car at the very back of the lot so you have to walk in to work, to the grocery, to your children's school. Move. Move. Move . . . it to lose it.

I recall one woman from a group at Aiken who lamented, "Why, Tamara, I used to hike, and Jeez, I miss it." Miss it? Well of course, she had to be missing it. This woman had been working a new job, putting in long hours each week, and was taking care of a household and a family, and she felt terribly guilty about stealing even a few hours on a weekend for herself. Even though her obesity was killing her, she was blind to the fact that her hikes had been essential.

I never join pity parties in Fat Chat sessions. Someone may come in with a litany of horror stories that all happened in the previous week. Yes, she needs to share them, and yes, she gets all of the group's support. But pity? No way. Don't go looking for it in your own life, either. Look for that push toward good health, that bit of support, someone to share a walk or class, but don't invite anyone on your journey who will pity you. "Poor you. Poor me." This is not what you need.

I had and I still have every excuse in the book for regaining every last one of those 100 pounds, plus more. I'll bet you have a million reasons why being fat scares you to death, but taking that first, second, or yet another step to good health is even more frightening.

Seven years ago, as I took my own first steps back here in the U.S.A. and into what I discovered to be my own brave, new world, my husband's family preferred to stay at their own pity party. They were so threatened by the journey I had begun that I couldn't wait to get out and back on my own. Finally, we got our assignment to head back South. This time, Fort Gordon, Georgia, would be our home base.

Though housing had a big question mark alongside it, we put the four kids into our van and headed out. Finances, or should I say, our lack of them, made every step we took stressful. For a big military family like ours, money was always, always an issue, and when we first arrived at Fort Gordon, we actually slept in the van for several nights until the guest house was available. Eventually, we got our own place, but what happened in this transition was that my self-confidence waned, and along with it, my energy level took a nosedive. Old routines are so hard to break. My bike, which had been shipped back from Germany, lay unused, and I climbed back into the car for every errand during that summer and fall of 1993. Those spiderwebs I'm always tryin' to clear out of other people's minds now were growing wildly in my own.

Do you know what happened next? I began to worry about my weight and focus on those numbers on the scale. Then I started taking away my calories. Yet, if I hadn't fallen back into that trap, a real shame for me, I might not have discovered the most valuable lesson of all for you.

I think you may have to be willing to settle for the messiness of experience. That may be what we mean by life.

DANIEL J. BOORSTIN

6

To Lose 100 Pounds . . .

"I Discovered That Small Changes Are Always Better than None"

The Person

The only way to change one's body weight is to begin a lifelong series of new habits.

Dr. Jules Hirsch

On a Trail in Brookdale Park, Montclair, New Jersey:

Tamara and I are walking faster than I usually do in this county park two blocks from my house. On average, a complete, door-to-door circuit for me around the park's perimeter takes about an hour. Today, keeping up with Tamara will shorten the hike for sure. All the same, we are having fun. She wants to do part of the walk backward, in fact. "You use different muscles walking backward," she explains.

"Oh really," I reply. "Sounds difficult. Do we have to?"

"Come on. It'll feel good." So, we turn around, and she keeps right on marching up an incline near the rose garden but going backward. I follow her lead and soon realize that this position does use different leg muscles, and it also forces me to twist my head, neck, and upper torso around. I'm trying to make sure that I don't run into a tree or person on the path, but the movement does feel great in my neck and shoulders, which become stiff when I sit too long at the computer. Who would have thought!!!

"You've got to have fun. Understand this," Tamara says: "Far too many weight-loss programs equate success with loss. Their standard of success is built only on your loss of pounds and not on your gaining knowledge and new habits. Eating as well as exercising become unnatural or unnaturally rooted in feeling bad about yourself. This should be your mantra: 'I am a can-do person. I am a can-do person. I am a can-do person.'"

"Hey, slow up," I plead, wondering how she can keep talking while walking so fast, still backward. "I'm not so sure I can do this."

"Let's go, girl. I know you can."

Do you realize that I've lost ten pounds since I began my chat sessions with Tamara? And I'm not even a regular member of Fat Chat. I didn't need to lose 100 pounds, but I had always dreamed of dropping 15 stubborn ones. Before I began researching Tamara Hill and her Fat Chat, I weighed 140 pounds, and at 5′3″, I had put getting into better shape on my to-do list.

So, you're wondering how I have managed to drop ten pounds in about five months? Easy. No sweat. The changes have been small and minimally intrusive, just as Tamara says.

Back in March, Tamara had asked me, "Do you eat breakfast?"

"Well, no," I answered. "I prefer to stick to coffee until lunch. I'm just not that hungry in the morning, so why waste the calories?"

The first thing that Tamara suggested was that I eat breakfast in the morning, even just a piece of fruit, to fuel my body and speed up my metabolism earlier in my day. Breakfast, I learned, would move my body out of the starvation mode that it had adopted during sleep.

"OK." So, I started the routine of eating a bowl of cereal within the first forty-five minutes after climbing out of bed. Slowly, subtly, I could feel myself hungrier later in midmorning. Then, I'd slice a piece of fruit to satisfy my hunger. This was new. This was different. One morning, after pulling the scale out from behind the laundry basket where I keep it hidden, I discovered that I had lost four pounds.

"Do you drink water?" Tamara queried.

"Well, not much," I replied. "I know I should, but I'm just not that thirsty."

"Your body is like an ocean," she said. "It's made up of 60 to 70 percent fluid. It needs water. Your muscles need water. Your brain works better with fluid, and so does your digestive system. Most people don't get enough water. They walk around dehydrated. I can feel my body flagging when I don't get enough plain old water. When you are heavier, like so many of my Fat Chat participants, you need even more water. If I drink a half cup of water during a class when I've been exerting myself, 95 percent of that water is dispersed throughout my body within fifteen minutes. If I relied on sports drinks or sugary sodas, fifteen minutes later, my stomach would still be trying to digest the fluids even though my body was crying out for hydration." Her advice: "Do me a favor," she said, "drink a glass of water whenever you pass your kitchen sink."

So, I began drinking more water. I put a couple of bottles of water next to my computer so I could sip while working. As a result, now I recognize signs of thirst. On occasion, I can gulp down an entire 16-ounce bottle within minutes. After a walk around the park or a game of tennis with my friend, Sue, I'm dying of thirst, something that had rarely ever happened before. Like the magic weight-loss potion Tamara denounces as nonexistent, drinking more water may be a rather miraculous ingredient in any new lifestyle.

"Take small steps," she says. A few little steps each day can result in great health benefits. "So many people are defeated before they even begin because they believe that big changes are the only way to get healthy. That's bull. The choices you make all the time can be small: white cake instead of the double-fudge version, a bag of fat-free Starburst candy instead of a Snickers bar, or a bottle of water versus that sugar soda. I don't circle the mall for fifteen minutes looking for a parking spot closest to the door; I park out in the boonies and walk. I use the stairs instead of elevators or escalators. I have hidden the TV remote control so I have to get up off the couch in my house to change the channels on the television and on the stereo, too. I carry in one bag of groceries at a time to increase the number of calorie-burning trips from the kitchen to the car and to incorporate exercise into my everyday life.

"If you want it, you can get exercise anyplace, all day long. I started by walking in my neighborhood with my kids after supper. You can be creative about finding time, because there are 1,440 minutes in a day. Small baby steps are all that you need to take. That's why when people say to me, 'Oooooh, I just don't have thirty minutes to exercise,' I say, 'Hah. Who the heck said you needed thirty minutes?'

"Think about it: You start moving. Ten minutes are up, and your body's metabolic rate is higher as a result. It will stay up there for a certain period of time, a period that varies for every individual, but during this higher sustained metabolic rate, you burn calories at a higher rate. This metabolic speedup could last up to an hour or two before it comes back down. If you do another ten minutes of exercise a little later in the day, you heighten your rate all over again for another hour. So, theoretically, if you do just one workout a day, you've heightened your rate only once."

> *The great mistake is doing nothing at all because you could only do a little—enough littles add up to a lot.*
>
> DON ASLETT,
> *HOW TO HAVE A 48-HOUR DAY*

"As we hike back up Cooper Avenue," she says, "you've got to think: Can I do this for the rest of my life without feeling deprived?" She declares, "Weight loss is easy. You can pay your money and have someone starve you. Almost everyone will tell you this. When you reach those three numbers on the scale—numbers that were predetermined by someone else, not necessarily you, you're out the door. Then, what happens?"

"What?" I ask.

"If you are like most people, you gain it back."

We are almost to the top of the hill near Park Street when she suggests, "Let's go to the Dunkin' Donuts uptown. I'm dying to have a muffin . . . one of those banana fat-free kind." She's persuasive: "Mmmmmm, don't you want one?"

Venturing into Dunkin' Donuts has never been easier. As she demonstrates so clearly, you don't have to give up your life in order to gain control over your health. You can have your cake, or should I say muffin, and eat it too. Just make wise choices so the consequences of your actions are ones that allow you to live a long and healthy life.

Becoming more fit can take twenty years off a person's chronological age.

Dr. Steven Blair, Cooper Institute
of Aerobics Research

The Program

James Brown's Boss Radio Station WAAW, 94.7:

Susan Mayberry is the host of Boss Radio's morning "Chit Chat" show which broadcasts from an old, semirenovated storefront building in Augusta's changing downtown area. Joined by Stacey Brown, the daughter-in-law of legendary rocker James Brown, who owns the station, Susan has scheduled Tamara for a Wednesday-morning show so we can discuss her Fat Chat program with listeners.

Backstage, we speak with the producer and other guests who will follow our appearance. The broadcasting studio sits in the corner of the building on the first floor, right at street level, and an expanse of windows allows passers to watch the action. A bar complete with stools surrounds Susan, who is in the hot seat as the host. Stacey sits up at the counter, alongside Tamara and me, where she reads her take on the day's news events and adds a bit of commentary here and there and in between tunes. This is fun, I think. No wonder some radio shows sound so relaxed. They are relaxed, and this morning is just like one of Tamara's ongoing chat sessions.

After a flurry of on-air introductions and welcomes, Tamara describes pieces of her program. "Susan, when I was 250 pounds, I had no place to go and no real understanding of where to begin. I needed someone—someone like *me!*—to help me stay motivated and to give me positive insight into how I could get healthy. Fat Chat combines mind, body, and spirit, and we meet each week. At the hospital, where the program first began, sessions run for sixteen weeks, but I've modified it for Powerhouse Gym and Fitness Works so that four months aren't really necessary. New people are always coming in and old friends return to get refreshed. In the first session, I distribute glossy folders with informational handouts and assignments. We start with questions to ease people into examining their lives. I ask, "Where are you now?" Then, we go over questions like, "Have you always been heavy?" and

"When did you first start gaining weight?" Really, I've got fifty or sixty great questions that will lead us all into a new awareness. One of my work sheets asks, "How do you like to exercise—By yourself? With a friend? With your husband? Outdoors? What time of day?"

"This is the thing," she explains, "most gyms and fitness clubs take your membership money, and they may set you up with a routine, but you are usually set up to fail. When you say the word *exercise* to a lot of women, they go, 'Whooooaaa, too scary for me.' They picture thin people in leotards somewhere between the ages of eighteen and twenty-one. Who wouldn't cringe at that image? I did. But that was before I understood how important it is to move my body and, eventually, how good movement makes me feel.

"My God, girls, I thought I was going to die in the first aerobic classes I took. Seriously, no kidding. I'm tellin' you, I had asthma and said to myself, 'Oh Lord, this is just too much for me.' Yet, the steps I started taking way back seven years ago were never awful. My journey has been wonderful, glorious, and even when it was hard, I knew I could never turn back."

A fellow from US Too!, a prostate-cancer survivor group in Augusta, is seated behind us on a couch near the window. He is scheduled to be interviewed following us, and I notice that his interest in Tamara's ideas has peaked as her energy level has risen.

"I firmly believe that the most sensible and healthiest approach to lose weight and manage it long-term is to make small adjustments in your habits and routines," Tamara says. "Your lifestyle is made up of all your habits and routines. These habits that you've formed, both good and bad, are in response to your everyday living. Your habits are formed by repetition and following the same routines day after day. Your habits, good or bad, are your way of responding to things and doing things. Many times, the pressures of daily life force us into unhealthy habits."

If you sit around or, worse yet, go to sleep after eating a large load of fat, it's the fat cells that are activated. It takes them only four to eight hours to absorb most of the fat you've taken in.

RONALD M. KRAUSS, M.D., UNIVERSITY
OF CALIFORNIA AT BERKELEY, CHAIR OF
THE NUTRITION COMMITTEE OF THE
AMERICAN HEART ASSOCIATION

Having watched Tamara's pressured life as a single mother up close, I know intimately that she understands the urge to eat fast foods, to stop by the Dunkin' Donuts, the McDonald's, the KFC. After all, she's busy, and biologically, human beings are programmed to eat this stuff because it's high in fats and sugars. Kelly Brownell, a Yale professor and leading obesity researcher, notes that "the pressure to take responsibility for what we eat is staggering," and adds, "Is there anyone in America who doesn't know that we should weigh less and exercise more?" As Brownell explains, "Animals and people evolved in an environment where food was scarce and calorie expenditures were high. Under those conditions, being programmed to eat high-calorie food is adaptive. Those ancient genes would not be a problem if the environment weren't so damaging."

The "toxic environment" Brownell describes is "a combination of food and lack of physical activity, the remote control, video games, the automobile, television, and to some extent the computer." This obesity specialist even asks, "Is Joe Camel any different from Ronald McDonald? One could claim that both encourage children to adopt habits that could be bad for their health."

We live in a fast-paced society that has traded nutrition for convenience, encouraging fast foods, takeout, microwave meals, snack foods, and other components of a high-fat diet. . . . But the environment isn't the only factor. New research suggests that brain chemistry can dictate a strong craving for fatty foods—a physiological "fat tooth."

JOSEPH C. PISCATELLA,
CONTROLLING YOUR FAT TOOTH

Fat Chat is designed to help change habits, Tamara explains during her segment. "Keep in mind that your habits are learned behaviors and that you have a choice to continue or to change them. Remember also that habits are very powerful and sometimes can be very hard to break. Don't expect to change habits overnight. Changing habits is a time-consuming process. Try making small, manageable changes that you can live with for the rest of your life.

"Your habits also reflect your attitude, and your attitude is key. You must tell yourself that you are a stronger, more in-control person now.

You must see yourself as a person who enjoys change and likes challenges. If you adjust your routines, habits, attitudes, and behaviors in your lifestyle," she says, to everyone in the Augusta listening area who is tuned in today, "you can reduce the risk of health problems and gain control of your weight." Do they listen? Yes. If you are within earshot of this formerly fat, energetic missionary, you can't help but get excited about the possibilities.

"I want to bring you to the end of a tunnel," Tamara announces. "I want to turn on the light. Let's talk about nutrition. Let's talk about exercise. Let's talk common sense and about feeling better every day. Let's talk about the only real reason anyone should want to lose weight: health. I learned a lesson, and anyone can. New habits—small changes—can become as easy as brushing your teeth or combing your hair. The biochemicals released by your brain will give you the right rush of energy. Your body, fat or thin, needs this relief. Just keep thinking: If I can do it, so can you!"

Susan Mayberry, Stacey Brown, and I can't help but smile at this woman. Behind us, waiting near the windows, is prostate-cancer survivor J. W. Solum, the chapter coordinator for us, Too! He jumps to his feet as Susan signs us off the air and goes to a prerecorded commercial.

Solum rushes over to Tamara and says, "This is so exciting. My wife really needs you. I'm going to tell her all about this Fat Chat, but I'm worried about her knees."

"I'm teaching water aerobics now," Tamara responds quickly. "Would she be interested in those classes? There is a way for everyone to feel better."

Tamara's Journey . . . in Her Own Words

People often fight themselves over weight loss. It is, as recent brain research indicates, a futile and useless fight, for humans love food. The search for the edible and the delicious is constant in history.

ROBERT ORNSTEIN AND RICHARD
F. THOMPSON, *THE AMAZING BRAIN*

At Her Home on Linderwood Drive:

Back at Fort Gordon, I was back into my old lifestyle. On-base housing, taking care of my kids, I wasn't really doing anything. The bike riding had ended. I was busy trying to move my family into a new home and get us all settled, so I spent all my time either in the car or in the house. This was the summer and fall of 1993, and I realized that my life had been so much different in Germany, but I didn't seem to be able to do anything about it.

There was no time for me. Though I'd think, "I've got to do something here," each day I'd get up and stick with the same old routine. I started gaining a little weight back, maybe ten to fifteen pounds, which was not a lot but was significant just the same. I kept thinking that there had to be something better in my life, but the only thing I could see to do was to take away some of my food. This was definitely the American way to get control over your body. The other thing I discovered by January of 1994 was that I didn't have the energetic feeling I had found in Europe.

"What am I doing here?" I asked myself. I was starving myself and taking away calories. I wasn't moving my body very much. I wasn't taking care of me at all. What had happened to my three principles? Jeez.

I called the gym on Fort Gordon. Yep. That's what I did. Other wives did go to these gyms, but mostly to aerobics classes, which is where I started. I remember my first class. This cute little gal led us. She was short and muscular, obviously had had no babies, and was way younger than me. "Fancy this," I thought. I was so out of place, but you know what? I decided not to give a heck. I was there for me. Classes were held in the evenings at 6:30 P.M., so my ex-husband would come in the door from his duty, and I'd go out to the gym, where I knew that I belonged. We did floor exercises and aerobic routines but no weight lifting. The steps were hard, and I thought I'd never get them, but I also thought, "This is OK."

At the end of the first week of attending classes every single day, I thought I was going to die. I just knew I was going to die because I felt so bad. I even started having physical problems because I had never done this type of activity in my life. Shinsplints, swollen ankles plagued me. I could hardly walk without crying and wanted to cringe because my legs hurt so much. It was a perfect opportunity for me to quit, but

I kept thinking, "This I can do. This is just my body fighting me. This is just me learning how to move my body." Back then, I hadn't read anything about the effect of exercise on a body out of condition and overweight. I decided that I had to take the good and the bad.

Are you familiar with shinsplints? I'm tellin' you, the pains in the front of my lower legs were excruciating. It's a condition that occurs as a result of repeated straining of the muscles attached to the shin bones. The muscles actually swell and press on the blood vessels, and though the symptoms are supposed to disappear within a week or two, mine didn't. Shinsplints can also indicate stress fractures, so I went to a sports medicine specialist on base. No, I didn't feel funny going to him, because my mind was set: Gol' dang it, I wanted to keep on exercising, and somebody had to help me. I also wanted to make sure there was nothing orthopedically or seriously wrong, because I didn't want to hurt myself.

"Ms. Hill," he said to me, "there is nothing wrong with your body. It is just telling you in unpleasant terms that you have let these muscles deteriorate. You haven't been working them." He sent me on my way with advice about taking a few days off and instructions for how to ice the injured areas and follow up with heat packs.

Giving up would have been so much easier than sticking with the exercise classes. Some days, I'd be in such agony that I had to wrap up my ankles before class. They'd be so swollen, and yet there was no particular reason for the swelling except that I was out of shape. Neglect . . . that's what had caused my body's violent reaction to exercise.

You've got to know that this might happen to you, too. Some of my new friends in class thought I was nuts to continue. Occasionally, at the end of the period, I'd be in tears sitting there on a step, unwrapping my ankles. "You are a crazy woman," someone said to me once, though not in a mean way. Most people were supportive, and I know if you search hard enough, you can find the same kind of support and excitement that I did.

It is said that if you could put the benefits of exercise in a pill, it would be the single most prescribed medication in the world. . . . One way to make something a habit is to have the same environment, the same situation every time you exercise.

KERRY COURNEYA, PH.D., ASSISTANT
PROFESSOR, UNIVERSITY OF CALGARY

You know what happened next? The shinsplints disappeared. The ankles stopped swelling. I became stronger and stronger. My bones, my muscles, my ligaments, everything about my body had been so weak that my muscles couldn't even support my own frame. I had to work through this stage, simply and slowly. There was no quick fix. It didn't happen overnight. Three minutes a day of breathing in and out didn't get me into shape. I didn't pray for a miracle and have the weight disappear and my body become strong with defined muscles.

I graduated from aerobics to a step aerobics class at the gym. Too many women use the excuse of their children for not being able to work out, but I always see this as their way of being iffy about making the commitment to good health. I won't let them, because I never used my kids this way. If my ex-husband wanted to play racquetball and we both went to the gym at the same time, we would pack toys. Right there in front of the aerobics room, there was a little table at which my kids would sit and play.

You know, girl, my roots of real wellness go back to that gym and the track, too. I started walking the track with my kids because we couldn't afford to hire a sitter. In my mind, there was a progression in which I saw myself getting healthier and healthier, stronger and stronger. This is no lie. I had an old, two-seater stroller, and the track at Fort Gordon has a clay base. I would take that stroller and push it through the clay with my two littlest ones in it. Little Clifford would walk alongside a lot of times, but I must have been pushing at least fifty to sixty pounds. Sometimes, my son Jeremy would come along, too. I'd push that sucker—the stroller, that is—almost every day, and when Cassandra and Kaye wanted to climb out, I'd find myself lugging them in and out.

Walking the track together gave me great opportunities for talking with my children. I will never forget some of those conversations. "Why do we have to walk, Mommy?" one or the other would ask. "This is fun, but it's also working our heart muscles; this is what we do to stay healthy," I'd explain. I wanted my kids to understand that exercise is essential and part of their lives. Still, I never say to my Fat Chat gals, "Monday, Tuesday, Wednesday, Thursday . . . I want to see you in class every day." Absolutely not; you have to do what's good for you. I ask people, "What are you comfortable with? Where do you want to start? With a walk? Do you have a dog?" Some women who have dogs may even be paying someone else to walk it.

There are basically two, possibly three, conditions under which
physical activity becomes an established part of one's life. The first,
and most reliable, is when you find something that contributes to
your self-concept and builds your self-esteem. . . . The second con-
dition is governed by the pleasure principle. If you find something
that gives you tremendous physical pleasure and a feeling of well-
being, then you are likely to stick with it. . . . The third condition
has to do with your work. Many people find that taking time to
be alone, walking or gently jogging, is their most creative time.

MARTIN KATAHN, PH.D., *ONE MEAL*
AT A TIME

By the fall of 1994, I started to think about becoming an aerobics
instructor. I was still out there on the track. I was still going to the
gym. People on base had heard my story, heard about my kids, and
heard about how much weight I had lost. They wanted to hear more.
So, I approached one of my instructors, Barbara, who is someone I
greatly admired, and asked, "Where do I go to get certified? What do
I do? How can I start this process?"

7

To Lose 100 Pounds . . .

"I Began to Love How My Body Moved"

The Person

Most of us are overwhelmed with information—but are starved for true knowledge.

John Chaffee, Ph.D., *The Thinker's Way: 8 Steps to a Richer Life*

From the Piles of Paper in My Upper Montclair Office:

Tamara is a long-standing member of the National Weight Control Registry (NWCR) based at the University of Pittsburgh Medical Center. She is especially proud of this particular affiliation. She faxes me correspondence from an NWCR representative, Rena R. Wing, Ph.D, as well as a *Reader's Digest* article and clippings from the journals of the American Society for Clinical Nutrition and American Dietetic Association. She tells me her official registration number with excitement. "I was one of the beginning members back in 1994," she says. "These people are just so great and have been a resource for me, providing a place to talk, to discover what others like me are doing."

As part of this ongoing study which now includes more than two thousand women and men who have successfully lost a minimum of thirty pounds and kept the weight off for longer than six years, Tamara is one of an elite group. She attests, "I lost 100 pounds, and not only have I kept it off but also I'm probably the only one who has gone on to start my own hospital-based program. No one else is out there doing what I'm doing."

What this team of researchers from the University of Pittsburgh and the University of Colorado have shown, and what makes Tamara so excited about being part of the program, is that anyone can break out of the obesity trap once and for all. Dr. Wing, a psychologist with the NWCR, says that even yo-yo dieting "does not make it more dangerous or difficult to lose weight." Forget about that genetic excuse, as well. In fact, a majority of the most successful NWCR losers had one and even two parents who were overweight, which underscores the notion that your biology isn't necessarily your destiny. The study also supports many of Tamara's own conclusions which have been incorporated into her Fat Chat philosophy.

"Read through this material," she urges me. "You are not going to believe it. This is the largest study of its kind in the United States and confirms so much of what I say every day. Girl, just wait till you see what it says. I know I'm right."

So, I start to pore through the paperwork, and after months of listening to Tamara's voice and her Fat Chat followers, it's nice to see her success placed into a larger context. This is serious stuff. "Congratulations," writes Dr. Wing, lead investigator of the research team. "Thank you for working with us over the past several years." Even more impressive, the materials show that Tamara and her fellow participants have provided data for presentations to the American Association for the Study of Obesity, the Society of Behavioral Medicine, and the American College of Sports Medicine, among others.

Here's a sampling of the findings:

• Nearly 77 percent of a sample of 629 women and 155 men in one NWCR analysis reported that a triggering event or incident had preceded their successful weight loss. In an article titled "A Descriptive Study of Individuals Successful at Long-Term Maintenance of Substantial Weight Loss" published in the *American Journal of Clinical Nutrition*, authors Mary Lou Klem, Rena Wing, and others explain that men and women both reported these turning points that Tamara has described so often. Some, mostly men, pointed to a medical trigger such as varicose veins, sleep apnea, low-back pain, fatigue, or aching legs. Others, particularly women, told of emotional issues that changed their lives. "My husband left me, and my lawyer told me it was because I was fat," one woman wrote. "My mother had to die of obesity-related complications," Tamara says, "and even then, I might never have started my journey to wellness if it hadn't been for my poppa."

• There is no perfect way to good health, and a very personalized plan worked the best. To be successful, reports Klem, a senior research fellow at the University of Pittsburgh School of Medicine, the dieters "tried many things to lose weight and finally found a combination that worked for them." A "great diversity in strategies suggests that individuals may be more likely to lose weight and maintain the loss if, rather than attempting to use one standard set of strategies, they selectively choose their means of restricting dietary intake and increasing activity level," the authors state. What didn't work were diet pills, surgery, or giving up favorite foods. "Just what I've said all along," Tamara points out. One woman incorporated black beans, something she loved, into a weight-loss program and dropped seventy pounds. Some people in the NWCR group needed the support of a formal program like Weight Watchers or Overeaters Anonymous, but 45 percent found the power within themselves, just the way Tamara did in Germany.

Movement burns up adrenaline and tension. Walking, jogging, biking, swimming, dancing, even karate will leave you feeling comfortably tired at first, then actually energized as you become practiced.

GEORGIA WITKIN, PH.D., *QUICK FIXES AND SMALL COMFORTS*

• Almost 100 percent changed their physical activity levels in some way. "Haven't I been saying all along, '*Move it to lose it*'?" Tamara insists. Again, not everybody in the NWCR registry is doing the same kinds of exercise or working at the same intensity. Whatever turned them on was the name of the successful game. Cycling, aerobics, walking, running, hiking, using a stair stepper, and swimming all showed up on questionnaires. Women were more likely to be walking or in aerobic dance classes, while men were into competitive sports or weight lifting. "I try to build fitness into my workday," one woman explained. "I walk rather than drive, and ride my bike as much as I can."

• Religious calorie counting or restriction was not the best way to go. According to 92 percent, "The strategy most frequently used" was to "limit intake of certain types of foods." Some cut down on meats and fried foods. Others learned how to read labels so they could monitor their high-fat and high-calorie foods.

• The "quick-fix" or "kill-yourself" philosophies were not helpful. Someone in the NWCR group said, "I had tried training programs that were way too strenuous for me. That only led to frustration and giving up." When asked to compare their success with previous failures, 82 percent said that they became "committed to making behavioral changes."

• Perhaps the most surprising support of what Tamara has been saying to me for nearly a year is that maintaining her loss of 100 pounds has not been difficult. Using a seven-point scale in which 1 represents "extremely easy" and 7 is "extremely hard," 30.3 percent of the NWCR study participants rated their everyday lives "easy," and 37.3 percent rated them "moderately easy." Only 32.4 percent of the 629 women and 155 men said it was extremely hard keeping the excess weight off.

"Didn't I tell you that my journey has been wonderful?" Tamara says later when we discuss the Pittsburgh-based study. "I remember thinking that I had to go, to learn, to listen, and to take in what the experts were saying, but I had to do it my way. Now my commitment to staying healthy is not a hardship. Not at all. Like the others in NWCR, I'm not feeling restricted or deprived. I built my own path, but I've enjoyed every step, even those times when I was physically hurting from sore muscles. I look forward to moving my body and to the classes I teach.

"Believe me, I've learned this important lesson: I move my body every day, and now my body looks forward to this. It's a relief. My brain needs the endorphins released during a workout. There is a mental high that comes when I'm moving. You need it. Everyone does. These biochemicals are released throughout your body, and you get a rush of energy."

*When you concentrate, your mind is like a spotlight, pouring
energy into a task and putting everything else in the dark
background. If an intrusive thought breaks out of its
compartment, the frontal lobe (of your brain) can pull the
spotlight back where it belongs.*

MARTIN GRODER, M.D., *BUSINESS
GAMES: HOW TO RECOGNIZE THE PLAYERS
AND DEAL WITH THEM*

Is Tamara the only one of these NWCR participants who seems to
be so much happier in general now? Not at all. Eighty-five percent of
the NWCR sample, as cited in the American Society for Clinical Nutrition article, echoed Tamara's sense of overall well-being. Was it hard
to stay healthy? No. Maintenance—no longer a dirty word—had
become a new way of living. Hundreds reported "improvements in general quality of life, level of energy, physical mobility, general mood,
self-confidence, and physical health."

The Program

Aurora Pavilion, Aiken Regional Medical Centers:

*At every moment, a woman makes a choice: between the state
of the queen and the state of the slave girl. In our natural
state, we are glorious beings. In the world of illusion, we are
lost and imprisoned, slaves to our appetites and our will to false
power. Our jailer is a three-headed monster: one head our past,
one our insecurity, and one our popular culture.*

MARIANNE WILLIAMSON,
A WOMAN'S WORTH

Stories spill out in Fat Chat sessions. Tonight the talk will eventually get around to exercise, which is on the agenda for both weeks
ten and eleven. *Find an Exercise That's Right for You*, Tamara's handout
proclaims. Another states, *Begin to Enjoy How Your Body Moves*.

"We are not here to talk about bulging biceps or rock-hard abs," Tamara tells the group this evening. Everyone laughs.

"What about looking good in a string bikini?" someone asks.

"Show us your muscles, Tamara!"

As a group, this class is proud of their teacher. A spirit of sharing and caring strengthens the connection and makes it easy to chat. "You don't want to see my muscles," she says.

"Oh, yes we do," someone to my right says. So, Tamara pushes up her T-shirt sleeve, smiles broadly, and makes a muscle for our benefit.

"You know," Ann says, "I had surgery once, and when the doctor talked to me about the stitches, he said, 'Well, you won't be able to wear a bikini for a while.' I said, 'That's fine, because I've never been able to wear a bikini.'" Ann explains, "I had severe chest pains and high blood pressure, so I've been coming here for more than a year for health reasons. I've got a heart condition, and the doctor was so concerned that he put me on a low-fat diet and told me to start exercising. So, I looked for an aerobics class and went, but only a couple of times. These skinny little 'things' would get up there in the front of class in their leotards and whoop, whoop, whoop it up with hands flying. I'd go home and feel blach, blecch. Why should I go, only to come home feeling bad about myself? Then, I saw an article about Fat Chat in the paper, and I came. I felt really good about myself. I had been here about a month, I think, when I told Tamara that I didn't want to do the step exercises on the step. She makes you feel that you can speak up like that. 'You do what you want,' she said to me."

Monique adds quietly, "When Tamara says, 'Stop if it causes you pain,' boy, can I stop quickly. I haven't moved in a month."

Ann, who obviously loves the freedom that Tamara grants to tailor routines to your own situation, continues her step saga. "So, at the beginning of that class, I was the only one who didn't go into the closet to pull out the step. I just did my routine on the floor. Then, another lady said, 'I want to do it on the floor, too,' And then another. I don't do anything that hurts me, and Tamara is so good about modifying the moves so they make us feel good. I had arthritis in my knee, so I couldn't squat without someone helping me back up. In fact, they'd have to help me go down, too." She laughs. "Now," she says, "I can go down and back up just like everyone else. I even showed my doctor. It's so much fun, and I enjoy it. But for me, the important part of Fat Chat is the feel-good part."

Tamara encourages her to go on. Ann relates, "I remember, when I went on medication for my cholesterol, I had a reaction. At the doctor's office, I had weighed 197, and I didn't think I looked that bad. But, all the way home, I kept saying to myself, 'Ann, do you know how close that is to 200? That's only 3 pounds away from 200.' I was almost 200 pounds! So, for a while, I tried that liquid stuff to lose weight. Then, one day, I mentioned it to my gynecologist and pointed out that some hospitals were even recommending it in their weight-loss programs, so it must be OK. He looked at me from across his desk, leaned back in his chair, and said, 'I don't recommend that at all. Not at all.'"

"Doctors love me," Tamara says, smiling.

"You sound just like me," Linda says in response to Ann's tale of the scale. "This time last year, I was up to 198. Those quick-fix remedies go against everything we've been learning here, though."

Tamara agrees.

Ann wants to share another story with the group about a dramatic quick-fix failure. "I had these next-door neighbors who were really big people. Fat people with big bones," she says.

"I used to be a big person just like that," Tamara reminds everyone.

Ann continues, "My neighbors both went on this liquid diet prescribed by a university health center, and during that time I saw them regularly at their house. Month by month, we went all through the Christmas season, and they got smaller and smaller. It was amazing because they had been so big, so fat and tall, if you know what I mean. They become the success stories for the weight-loss center. Then, after they went off their liquid diets, they began to get bigger and bigger and bigger again." She concludes, "I don't think these centers go back to check on their success stories enough." she says.

A chorus of voices agree, "They don't."

"That reminds me of when my husband and I were dating," Peggy says. "When he was a baby, his mother always believed that being fat meant being healthy. She always felt better when she could see him eating. All three of her kids were big, but when my husband went to college and was then out on his own, he lost 100 pounds and didn't do it the healthy way. He would work overtime, eat nothing more than a pack of crackers or a diet soda all day, and then play tennis. After he lost the weight, he was sick for the next six months, which is when I met him. He still had a pair of his bigggggg—and I mean really big—pants, which I discovered by accident. One day when he was out of town and I was supposed to be taking care of his little dog, I went to his townhouse, and going upstairs, I almost died. Seriously. Suspended from the ceiling were these pants which scared me to death because I thought they were a person. Oooooh, I couldn't believe how huge they were."

This strikes a chord with Ann, who recounts, "My grandmother was a seamstress who used to make everything for us, her grandchildren. At her house one day, I went into the front bedroom which she used as a workroom. There on the wall, she had pinned up a pair of men's pants that were at least five feet wide." Gesturing with her arms, she says, "I'm not kidding." She continues, "Well, I said, 'Wooooo. Whose pants are they?' My grandmother explained that they belonged to a man named Mr. Roberts; she made all his clothing. I said, 'Is he really that big?' and she answered, 'Unh huh.' And then I asked her, 'Well, why do you pin them up onto the wall like that?' And she said, 'Why, I don't know. I just got into a crazzzeee mood.'

"I can remember thinking," Ann recalls, "How could anybody be that big and be able to breathe and live? Mr. Roberts drove a pickup truck, and anytime you saw him go by in the truck, it would be leaning to one side. The springs on the driver's side were all gone."

Honest chat about fat, depression, and power continues. "An average person like Mr. Roberts," Tamara observes, "wants the directions to good health spelled out exactly. Or he may want a pill because he doesn't think he has the power within himself. I keep right on saying that until you take back your own power, you aren't going to feel confident. It's got to come from here," she says, "and here," holding one hand over her heart and one over her head. "You are in total control over your own life, and learning this is what this group is all about."

"Yeah, well, that's pretty challenging," Monique says.

"Nobody said it wasn't going to be challenging," Tamara answers quickly. Then, a quiet settles over the group. Tamara lets her words hang in the air for a second. Timing is everything, and she knows how to command attention with her silence. After all the casual chatting about obesity, the comfort level shifts slightly. Using the pause to change the course of conversation, she says, "Now, I want to help you with an exercise program that will work for each of you. You don't have to come to my classes. You've just got to do whatever it takes to get you up and moving. Linda, what do you do for exercise?"

"I park in the back of the parking lot at school and walk," says Linda, who has gone back to college. "When I have a ton of books in my backpack, this is really helpful. I do it twice a day."

"She wasn't doing this before," Tamara says to the rest of the group. "She was taking the easy way out." She asks Linda, "Has it helped?"

"Yes, it's helped a lot," she affirms, prompting further testimony.

"I'm just not motivated to exercise on my own," Monique says. "But Peggy and I are a team when we walk together early in the morning. I've also been wanting to get into the water now that the seasons are changing."

"Think of regular exercise as the greatest gift you can give yourself," Tamara tells the group. "It is the gift of better health for the rest of your life. Your journey toward fitness begins with tiny steps. Starting slowly, make small, manageable changes, and progress gradually. Savor your accomplishments as you get healthier. Don't concentrate on outward appearances. The more you move your body, the more calories you will burn. You say you don't have time to exercise, but you will almost always find time for the things that are important to you. So, if you make exercise a priority in your everyday life, you will find time to do it and begin liking it."

"Oh, I know what you mean," Ann says.

"Ask yourself some important questions," Tamara advises:

- "How's your endurance level? Do you huff and puff when going up and down stairs?
- "How's your flexibility? When you bend over, do you need help to get back up?
- "How many excuses do you have? Do you feel that you should exercise but you really don't have the time, the energy, or the equipment?"

An early morning walk is a blessing for the whole day.

HENRY DAVID THOREAU

Glancing down at the sheet of ideas Tamara has put together, I realize that chatting, sharing, and caring about each other for an hour on a weekday evening makes her prescription so much easier to take. She asks all of us to follow five guidelines:

- Be creative about finding time to exercise.
- Find people we like to exercise with.
- Set realistic exercise goals.
- Find an exercise that we truly enjoy doing, so that we will continue doing it for the rest of our lives.
- Stay away from people or places that make us feel uncomfortable when we are exercising.

Tamara's Journey . . . in Her Own Words

Until one is committed, there is hesitating, the chance to draw back, always ineffectiveness. . . . The moment one definitely commits oneself, Providence moves too. All sorts of things occur to help one, that would never have otherwise occurred. A whole stream of events issues from the decision, raising in one's favor all manner of unforeseen incidents and material assistance which no man could have dreamed would come his way.

GOETHE

In Her Van on the Way Home from a Class:

My friend Barbara, who still lives here in Augusta and was one of my favorite aerobics instructors, was so helpful and so supportive of my journey. I admire her tremendously and enjoyed every minute of her classes. On Fort Gordon, I began to study with Barbara there at the gym, which was formally known as Fitness Center #6. Carmen, another gal, had also set this certification process as one of her goals, so the three of us would read, study, and work out together.

I tackled aerobics first and got a copy of the curriculum which is in book form. To pass the Aerobics and Fitness Association of America (AFAA) test, one requirement is to do what's called a practical, in which you get up and demonstrate how you would conduct a class. There's a written part to the exam along with this practical part, and I had to go to Atlanta for a full day of testing. Barbara, Carmen, and a few of the other gals from gym #6 drove up together. It was fun, and we had a good trip, but I failed the practical that first time and had to return. I had passed the written, so I was relieved not to have to redo the entire exam.

Meanwhile, I started teaching classes at the gym as I continued to study for other certifications. Many of the other gals who spent time in classes with me or encouraged me to stick with my mission are so proud of me now. Anyone who has watched me over the last seven years will tell you how far I have come and how I emerged. I was this big woman with massive flesh. I was just a housewife and a mother who never did anything for herself. Now I tell other women about self-love and acceptance of themselves. When I took the practical part of the AFAA exam a second time, I passed with flying colors.

Next, I started studying for the American Council on Exercise (ACE) certification. Using my brain like this was amazing to me. The ACE exam has no practical, but there are more than 175 questions, and it's a four-hour test. This organization really gets into bones, muscles, energy, and how food works in the body. While there are several multiple-choice answers that may be partially correct, you are supposed to find the one that is most correct. Whew. I'm tellin' you, it was hard, and I had to travel, and spend time and money, but I passed it the very first time. I'm in the process of renewing this certification right now, in fact. For all my certifications, I must attend seminars and workshops and have continuing-education credits to maintain my status and to keep ahead. I'm the kind of person now who would keep on studying even if I didn't have to, but this probably keeps the average instructor up to grade.

I also went on to pass the National Dance-Exercise Instructors Training Association (NDEITA) certification, the Aquatic Exercise Association (AEA) certification, and the American Red Cross Community Water Safety course in Aiken. Over there at Aiken Regional Medical Centers, we have a pool, and sometimes I'll sub for the water instructor. I love the water, I love to swim, and I want to be as diverse in my training as possible so I can offer people almost any kind of exercise. I also passed the American Heart Association's curriculum for cardiopulmonary resuscitation (CPR) to be an emergency cardiac-care provider.

As I was studying for all these exams and reading on my own, I began to wonder about muscles. Though I was stronger than I had ever been, I just didn't feel or look very muscular. There I was doing cardiopulmonary work all the time, but I knew that something was missing. I had started to work on step aerobics and was keeping up with my "run-walks," but late in 1994, I started to learn about weight training. I took it seriously as a woman because we all need to learn about osteoporosis, or bone disintegration, as we get older. While I didn't want to build bulky muscles, I discovered that by concentrating only on aerobic activities without any weight training at all, I might be hindering my body. The American College of Sports Medicine (ACSM) and the real experts on all this, say that you are getting only half the job done if you neglect to weight train. It's like trying to play tennis with your shoelaces untied.

So, I found a guy over at gym #6 to help me weight-train and whom I consider a real buddy to this day. Louis is a sergeant who used to come to my aerobics classes and has always been supportive. Through Louis, I learned how to lift weights in what is called the free-weight area. I didn't feel as if I belonged at first, and you can still count the women doing this on one hand in most gyms. This wasn't my area, but I thought, "What the heck?" Louis helped me out and would explain how much the different bars weighed and how to hold them and grip them, and the right hand position and form for the bench press. He taught me the basics, like a good trainer, and even now, years later, I still prefer to lift free weights as opposed to using machines or equipment. That's just me. That's why I always say that you can't base your own program on exactly what I do. If it's not your cup of tea, you aren't going to be able to stick with it.

Finally, another day arrived that I had only imagined in my dreams. From those slow and steady trips around the clay track with my kids in the double stroller, to my quarter-mile walks around the neighborhood, and on to what became a jogging routine, I graduated to my first official run. It was the 1994 Fort Gordon Autumn Classic 10 Kilometer race (about six miles). Out of 1,400 runners, mostly soldiers, I placed twelfth in my age category with a time of 59:43. I still have the printout of my time. Hardly any civilians entered, and even fewer wives, like me. These events were milestones for me. I didn't receive any trophy that first day, but I felt like a true winner just crossing the finish line.

This was my journey. I was doing all this for me, and I've participated in more races over the years which are always a lot of fun. You know, I think I've saved every number that was ever pinned on my shirt in a race. I knew back then, in 1994 and 1995, when all this was happening, that I could do anything I wanted if I set my mind on it. Unfortunately, my commitment to taking care of myself was intimidating to my husband. As I became more physically fit, he became more physically and verbally abusive. It was awful. Because he was still in the army, I'd have to call the military police, and I even pressed charges. He would get so mean that my personal life became a nightmare, a nightmare from which I had to escape.

8

To Lose 100 Pounds . . .

"I Knew for Sure That the Miracle Was in My Mind"

The Letters

> *Negative emotions such as chronic rage, hostility, and anger can contribute to serious problems. . . . We have a biochemical means of virtual instant communication between the mind and the emotions and any part of the body. These kinds of connections between brain and body explain why the mind has power over the body.*
>
> REED MOSKOWITZ, M.D.,
> *YOUR HEALING MIND*

B. Smith's Restaurant in New York City:

Tamara's mail makes a dramatic statement about her power. For a trip to New York, she has lugged piles and piles of rubber-banded letters from desperate or admiring women. "Look at these," she says to Agnes Birnbaum, our literary agent, and me. From a sack next to her chair at B. Smith's restaurant on Eighth Avenue, she pulls out several of the see-through plastic bags stuffed with envelopes. She reports, "I've received hundreds and hundreds of these amazing letters. More arrive every day. Yesterday I even spoke to a nun on the phone."

The diversity of the writers of these letters is reflected in their stationery. From clean business-white and typed correspondence, to pale pink, blue, and sunny yellow handwritten letters, to scrawled, one-line postcards, flower-motif notes, yellow legal-pad requests, and even little self-adhesive notes crammed into envelopes, the mail offers first-hand validation of several of the generalized statistics she's been citing. It's one thing to say that more than half of all Americans between ages twenty and seventy-four are overweight (one-fifth of that number are considered obese) and quite another matter when you see personal pleas from them asking why. These are real people, not numbers. "Obesity contributes to about 400,000 deaths a year," Tamara says. "If you are obese, you run a dramatically higher risk of developing diabetes, high blood pressure, high cholesterol, heart disease, or even cancer. If you are obese, you certainly do have a serious health problem, and these writers tell me how desperate, how sick, how scared they are. I have to help," she says.

"My God, Tamara," I say, "Can I borrow some of them? Will you let me read them?"

"Of course, girl," she replies. "Take them. Take them. That's why I brought them. I want you to read them and understand."

"But have you answered them?" I ask.

"No, not yet," she explains. "I've been crazed. The letters just keep pouring into my house, and I don't know where or how to start. I'm a single mother now, with five kids, trying to pay my bills and take care of my family. I open them, of course, but I can't afford to write back yet. I need this book so I can reach them."

Agnes and I nod approvingly because a book is exactly what we want, too.

"I'm tellin' you," she continues, "I am not a stranger to these people who feel compelled to sit down and write to me. They feel as if they know me because I'm no different from them. They can trust me. They are afraid.

"These letters come from everywhere," she adds. "Look. Look," she insists and then starts to read off postmarks: "Valrico, Florida; Sterling Heights, Michigan; Gaylord, Minnesota; Lee's Summit, Montana; Greenwood, Indiana; Syracuse, New York; South Deerfield, Massachusetts; Silver City, North Carolina; Cedar Crest, New Mexico; Florence, Kentucky. Every day, the mailman brings me more and more.

"You know," she confides, "people come up to me all the time to hug me because they feel a connection, an intimate connection, right away. I'm not threatening. I was fat. There's almost nothing about their lives that I don't already know. I am safe for them. In fact, so many write and say they have never written a letter to anyone like me before."

The thing women have to learn is that nobody gives you power. You just take it.

ROSEANNE ARNOLD

Articles in magazines such as *Prevention's Guide to Weight Loss* and *Ms. Fitness,* and especially the one in *McCall's* October 1997 issue, as well as other media coverage and appearances have worked like beacons bringing the letter writers into Tamara's life. She's been doing spots on WJBF News Channel 6 in Augusta, Georgia, as a fitness expert and was a guest on the *Montel Williams Show.* Local radio shows have invited her to spread the word, too, and Tamara has loved every second of her time on FOXIE 103 and WTHB 1550 AM in Augusta, as well as JOY 102 in Aiken and James Brown's Boss station WAAW 94.7. A frequent motivational speaker at local health fairs and corporations, she was a regional winner of the 1995 Milk FitWoman Award, sponsored by the Milk Industry Foundation and the Women's Sports Foundation. Meanwhile, her mission keeps growing, and followers clamor for more.

"Take them," she tells me again, passing packets of mail over to my side of the table. "You need to know these people so you will understand how important this mission is for me. They are looking for inspiration and for answers."

She tells us, "It feels so natural now to be reaching out like this to people on a national level. When I first started this journey, I was so self-oriented, going for my certifications and learning as much as I could about my own body. I was concerned only with losing the weight, getting healthy. I didn't have any idea of Tamara Hill inspiring anybody but herself. Then, as I progressed and began to speak in public about my own success story of fighting fat and getting fit, people would come up to me afterward. 'Let me shake your hand,' they'd say. Or, 'Can I give you a hug?' Or, 'God, you were so great up there, and I can't believe you were 100 pounds heavier.' These people would be impressed and inspired." She says, "I feel their struggle, their dilemmas, their depressions, their thoughts. It's not just me anymore. I am compelled to take this message of wellness to others."

The waitress has been patiently waiting at the side of our table to take our orders. "Are you ready?" she asks. We aren't, but we ask for the specials and suddenly, this young woman has joined our conversation. She is from Augusta, Georgia. "Isn't this amazing?" Agnes and I think. Not Tamara. It makes perfect sense to her that, like a magnet, she would draw someone from her town to serve her at a Manhattan restaurant thousands of miles from home.

"We're working on a book together," she tells the young lady before deciding on a cheeseburger. A cheeseburger? Of course.

And, yes, we are working on a book together. Though I had once believed that the last thing the publishing world needed was another book about weight loss and fitness, I've become convinced that something important has been missing from what already exists in the book marketplace, and that something is Tamara Hill.

When I worked for *Good Housekeeping, Ladies Home Journal,* and later *McCall's* magazine years ago, we would frequently run stories that tackled big sociological or psychological issues by tapping into our readers' opinions. If one thousand women responded to a topic, you could draw certain conclusions that made very interesting editorial copy. There are certainly formal approaches to polls, surveys, and studies that can make the data collected more legitimate and official, but sometimes our best stories were simply based on the fact that thousands of readers all used the same word or emotion to describe an issue close to their hearts and homes. As I began to read through the letters written to Tamara Hill, my mind clicked back to those old survey stories. What I had in my hands, in these letters, was an important and rather startling window to the puzzle of obesity. I also had the feeling that these letter writers had never been so completely honest with anyone else in their entire lives before—not with a close family member, not with a friend, and certainly not with a doctor or person in authority.

I spent days on a couch in my upstairs sitting room opening envelopes, rereading mail Tamara had already seen, trying to absorb the emotions and struggling to categorize letters. Hundreds of women wanted to join Fat Chat. No, let me make that thousands. In one line, one page, and six pages, they asked for support and understanding.

What I decided to do, to open new lines of communication for you, is to take a closer look at the common themes expressed in these letters. Keeping with the spirit of a chat session, the presentation of these writers' honesty may help you to be more honest with yourself.

I am so scared, they write. Fear is not an emotion commonly addressed in diet books or by fitness experts . . . at least not in the books I've read. Yet, fear prompts so many of these cries for help. Somehow, as Tamara always says, the "looking good" side of this horrible game still seems to overshadow the health issues. "Fear of Dying" just doesn't pop up easily as a chapter title or weight-loss program topic. The opposite is much more likely. In fact, the right to feel good about looking fat even shows up in the *New York Times*: a 5′5″ woman who weighs 300 pounds and is a board member of the National Association to Advance Fat Acceptance doesn't believe that obesity should be turned into a medical condition. Nevertheless, what I see when I read the mail I'm holding is an intense anxiety about medical conditions. (Each of the writers quoted here has graciously given permission to reproduce her words, but I decided to use initials instead of actual names to protect the writers' privacy.)

> Dear Tamara,
>
> I read your story in *Luxury Lifestyles Successful Slimming* magazine, and I had to write to you. You are where I want to be in my life. So, I am hoping you can help me get to where you are.
>
> I am almost thirty-four years old, and I don't want to die young. I am 5′4″ tall, and I weigh 250 pounds. In the last nine months, I have gone from 190 and a size 16 up to 250 and size 24. I have two children, a girl who will soon be thirteen and a boy who will be seventeen. I want to be around for my children, and I want to be healthy. I need help. I have a family history of heart disease and diabetes. I lost my father at the age of fourteen from heart failure along with complications of diabetes. My mother has high blood pressure and heart problems. I have always wanted to weigh between 140 and 150 pounds, but 100 pounds is a lot of weight to lose and then try to keep off. I am so ashamed of myself for letting my body get in such bad shape. I have a lot of guilt, and I feel sad, hurt, alone, and scared. I eat everything, and I eat just to be eating. I have no friends and very little family. I just keep to myself.—M. C.

I feel so alone, they say. The isolation M. C. addresses in her letter is discussed so often that I find myself wanting to pick up the phone and invite these people to walk in the park with me.

Dear Tamara,

I am writing to you concerning your inspiring story in *McCall's*. I, too, am about 100 pounds overweight. I am too embarrassed to find out just how much I do weigh! In an office full of much smaller women, I don't dare get involved in their incessant conversations about dieting and losing weight when my weight quite possibly would double any of theirs. You sound like just what I have been looking for because I need encouragement and understanding, not disapproval. Please send me information to create a plan to become a healthier, happier person.—K. H.

I'm in a bad relationship, they explain. As with Tamara's own story of a marriage spiraling downward, unbalanced relationships often contribute to these writers' problems.

Dear Tamara,

I know you probably get a lot of mail, but I decided to take a chance and write. I am miserable because I weigh 290 pounds at 5'6". I am separated from my husband, and when I do see him because we go out sometimes, he asks me when I am going to lose weight. He even made the comment that maybe he would come back to me if I could lose this weight. Part of me wants him back, and another part of me wants to go ahead with the divorce. He is very emotionally abusive. . . . —L. H.

Where do I start? they ask. L. H. continues . . .

Getting started on a diet or eating plan is so difficult because I am an emotional eater. I am very sensitive about people and the way I am treated by them. Presently, I am in college after taking nine years off. Sometimes I want to stop going because I can barely fit into the seats. The women at my college are attractive and thin.

Your story touched my life because it made me think about my situation. You are a very strong woman. Please give me any advice you have.—L. H.

In one study, when 555 women zapped their dietary fat in half for a year, they ended up feeling more vigorous, less anxious, and less depressed than they did when eating high-fat foods. They learned to chop fat through small group meetings.

GALE MALESKEY, *FIGHT FAT*

I am depressed, they admit. One of the stacks of opened letters in my office is labeled "Depressed," but it grows so high and the writers share so many characteristics with others that this category is almost all-encompassing. Sadness and self-disgust are everywhere. "Love self," one of those three principles repeated by Tamara almost every time she opens her mouth, is definitely missing from these women's lives. For years and decades, the letter writers have not believed that they are worthy of time off, time to exercise, special treats, or rewards.

Dear Tamara,

I just read the article in *McCall's* concerning your story of weight loss. It has really inspired me to do something—make a change in my life. Here is my story:

On February 28, 1970, I got married, and at that time I weighed 125 pounds. Now, almost twenty-eight years later, I weigh a whopping 230 pounds—more than 100 pounds too big. During this marriage, we produced four children. Like you, I feel as if I've given to the world for my whole married life. Now it's time for me. In October 1997, I turned fifty years old. For the last few years, especially the last five, I've been really depressed. I know it has a lot to do with myself and my weight. The way I look makes me feel bad physically and mentally. I have very low self-esteem. My children were my whole world when they were little. Now that they're grown (the last one is a senior in high school), I feel so alone. Yes, my husband is still around. He doesn't do anything for my feelings of loneliness and unhappiness. Oh, he tries, but I guess I just don't feel for him the way I used to. Anyway, that's a whole other story.

I want to be healthy. I feel as if I have no friends. All I do is work and go to the church, the grocery store, and the doctor when needed. I have no contact with old school friends. I hate where I live which is about fifteen miles outside of town. My husband will not even talk about moving into town because where we live now is where he grew up. This is where he is comfortable. I highly resent his being this way and have for years. My husband is a very negative person, but he doesn't realize this. He thinks he is one of the most positive people in the world. Yes, I realize that a large part of my problem with me is my husband. He has to be in control of everything, and most of the time, I feel as if I'm pressured and backed into a corner.

I just want to write or talk to someone who has been where I am now. I just need someone to confide in. Thanks for listening. —J. N.

I want to be healthy, they beg. Like so many of the Fat Chat women I met in Georgia and South Carolina, the writers feel a kinship with Tamara because she talks about diseases caused by obesity. These women know the details of diabetes, heart disease, and surgeries. Some even work in hospitals, where unpredictable schedules and junk-food binging are regular patterns.

Dear Tamara,

I'm nearly thirty-seven years old, married eleven years, with no children because of infertility caused by polycystic ovary disease. I'm hovering around 235–240 pounds since my gallbladder surgery in 1992. Diagnosed with Type II diabetes in 1987, I was placed on insulin in 1990, but I'm still not in good control. I work the second shift at a hospital and have difficulty eating at scheduled times because of my erratic waking and sleeping. Please help me.—N. M.

I've given everything to my family, they say. Very, very many are victims of their own good-natured willingness and natural inclination to keep right on giving to others until only feelings of emptiness remain, along with the excess pounds, of course. Mothers, just like J. N., author of a letter previously cited, have devoted decades of their lives to the care and feeding of their families, giving nothing substantial to themselves. Others describe lifestyles of caretaking that sound downright astounding to a mother of two, like me.

Dear Tamara,

I have never written about my weight to anyone before, but your before-and-after picture gives me hope. You are a great inspiration to me. I started another diet two weeks ago because I am 110 pounds overweight. I have three birth children, ages eight, five, and ten months. I also have four foster children, ages twelve, nine, eight, and seven. Now that six of the seven children are in school, I am ready for "me" time. I joined a club that offers day care. I faithfully have been doing step classes three times a week, but I have gained three pounds. I have a wonderful husband, but he is thin and doesn't understand what it is like to live in my body. I have been very overweight for fifteen years and I am now thirty years old. Please get back to me about your Fat Chat.—S. T.

Dear Ms. Hill,

I just read your story and loved it. It really comes at a good time for me. As a mother of six, including three birth children and three special needs, ranging in age from twenty-seven down to fourteen now, I just said those words of yours: "It has to be my time now!" I am about fifty pounds overweight, tired and just plain run-down. I know your way is the right way to go. As a matter of fact, tonight I am going to walk to the volleyball game instead of driving. I am also trying to join a women-only gym, but I will have to save a little bit more money before that is possible. Thanks for inspiring me. I know I can do it.—S. M.

Those pounds just kept on coming, they recall.

Dear Tamara,

I'll be dead at seventy-two. Your article in *McCall's* seemed as though it were written just for me. I am sixty-one years old, have always been active, raised eleven healthy, beautiful children, raised a garden, canned, baked, cooked everything from scratch, and gained a few pounds after every pregnancy which I never took off. After eleven children and fifty-some years, I was 217 pounds. Then, I kept adding a few more pounds every year, and now, at sixty-one, I am 230 pounds. I've just been diagnosed with Type II diabetes, and I take twenty milligrams of Prinivil for high blood pressure.

The ironic part of this is that I've been very health minded for many years, taking vitamins and minerals. I know how important it is to lose weight and to exercise, but I just cannot get my mind and body working. I moved from a small city to Omaha, a giant city, and I have no friends and haven't yet gotten acquainted in church activities because I have to work full-time. If I don't change my ways, I'll die.

Can I start a Fat Chat here so I will be involved in something to take my mind off feeling sorry for myself? Maybe by helping others, I will have a purpose in life. Any suggestions will be greatly appreciated.—Y. A.

I've tried all the diets, they explain. My sister-in-law Eileen used to conduct an obesity program in Pittsburgh, Pennsylvania. "You don't need to teach these people, as much as you need to inspire them," she cautions. "The women I worked with here in Pennsylvania knew the details of most every diet and fitness program better than I do. Many understood exactly what they had to do but just couldn't do it. Seriously, these individuals have tried everything." Eileen's words of warning about overteaching the technical aspects of weight loss hang there in the back of my mind for weeks. I start to count the number of letter writers who mention diet after diet after diet, from the newest ABC plan to last year's 1-2-3 variety. They have all been on a veritable roller coaster of weight loss and gain.

The premise of food-specific diets is that some foods have special properties that can cause weight loss. No food can.

Jane Kirby, R.D., *Dieting for Dummies*

Dear Tamara,

I was deeply touched by your strength and enthusiasm. I've been on a roller coaster physically and emotionally. I, too, am 100 pounds overweight. Before my second son was born in 1980, I had a model's body and felt so beautiful. Men lusted after and hounded me. I became pregnant in 1979 and gained 141 pounds, going from 140 to 280 in nine months. For seventeen and a half years, since 1980, I have struggled with weight and gallbladder problems. In 1988, I took charge of my health, joined an exercise group through a fitness center, and toned up considerably. Then in 1989, I went on a medically supervised diet and lost a lot of weight in six months. I felt so beautiful, felt appreciated, and men still lusted after me which deeply bothered me. I kept the weight off, but in 1995, I started to gain it back slowly. Now I'm close to 272 pounds, and I feel blah! I have been walking about two miles a day, but the seat on my bike broke because of my weight. I have been cutting back on my food intake, and I'm in a size 20. Even so, I feel as if I'm on an emotional roller coaster which affects both my weight and my life. What can I do to keep myself on a steady pace?

The only health problem I've had since 1980 is my gallbladder, and I will probably end up having surgery to have it removed. I'm almost forty years old, and I must get off this roller coaster. I want to be the next person to say, as you did, "I Lost 100 Pounds—and Got a Life!"—C. W.

The Program

Diets are prisons. . . . Diets do not take into consideration
physical hunger. They ignore the reasons for overeating and the
meaning of extra weight.

Jane R. Hirschmann and Lela
Zaphiropoulos, *Are You Hungry?*

My Third-Floor Office in Upper Montclair, New Jersey:

I call Tamara early on a Tuesday morning to describe my letter-reading experiences. I am exhausted and worried about everyone who has written to her.

"Wow," I say. "I want to start writing back to these people. They are all so wonderful and so in need of your energy and inspiration. Now I understand why you give hugs and emphasize sharing and caring in your sessions."

"I know. I know," she says. "I feel just terrible that I haven't been able to contact each one of them yet. But I feel worse about what society and the diet industry have done to them. Take a woman who has been about 130 pounds most of her life, maybe up until her child-bearing years. Then, she goes up to 180, 190, or even higher. Do you think that any diet, any expert, or any program should bring her quickly back down to 130? *No*, I don't think that it is necessary or even should be something to worry about. What we should be worrying about is how she is being bombarded every day, after day, after day, with negative feelings. I want to help this woman to start feeling good about herself, feeling good about moving, and changing some of her eating patterns so that her deepest feelings about herself will change. The miracle is right there in her own mind."

Tamara adds, "Even if you were able to get this person back down to her old 130 pounds or some ideal weight, would she be happy? Is her life suddenly going to be miraculously wonderful because of those three numbers? *No.* Will she be able to maintain that weight loss? Of course not. The miracle must begin in her mind because it's something she has to carry around with her every day for the rest of her life. She has to feel good. She can't feel depressed or deprived or bad because she will never be able to stay there. Diet specialists miss the whole point. Even I can see that missed connection, not just from my own experience but also from the letters and the people when I teach and speak. To lose 100 pounds, you have to find out who you are. Then, you have to understand what makes you tick."

Out at Fitness Works, in Edgefield, South Carolina, a series of Fat Chat sessions is coming to a close. "We've had a fantastic time," Tamara tells me. Owner Beth Martin is happy because several of the women have lost weight, and the aerobics classes are drawing up to twenty-five a night. Linda is down seventeen pounds; Carolyn, Misty, and Marge are happy, and Mary Anne has lost eight pounds. But it's not the weight that excites Tamara, as she makes clear: "These women have made the commitment to feeling better and have chosen to be enthusiastic no matter what happens. Every day, they are treating themselves in some small way, whether that means buying a size smaller pair of jeans or just celebrating by going for a walk on a beautiful sunny day. They have forgotten about trying to achieve a totally new shape and realize they don't need a new body. They've already got bodies worthy of respect."

The brain is the signature of one's wishes, desires, and actions . . . the more you exercise it, the more it develops . . . the instant you decide to take on a new subject, you have actually begun to expand your neuronal network.

RICHARD RESTAK, M.D.,
BRAIN RESEARCHER

In one of the recent sessions at Fitness Works, Tamara tackled the issue of procrastination. "When we don't want to expend the effort or energy, it's easier to say, 'I didn't have time to start today.' Or, we believe everything has got to be perfect in order to begin. Let's face it, you may never have the perfect combination of factors to begin your journey to wellness," she says. "I certainly didn't. My personal life was a mess."

Putting off what you know you should be doing can be a sign of fear, she explains. And why shouldn't you be afraid of failure? No one is more fearful than a fat person who has tried and failed in the dreadful diet game once, twice, or many times before. She poses questions to prompt discussion:

- Where else are you struggling?
- Has your energy increased?
- Are you still exercising?
- Are you thirstier now that you are drinking more water?
- Are you eating breakfast to start your body's engine?
- What are your nightmares?

She reminds anyone who needs assurance, "All change is scary. The changes in my own life during my journey were not small at all when I retrace my steps mentally. I took little steps, but in the end, I experienced enormous upheaval. Remember, you are not alone in your frustration, exhaustion, disappointment, and fear of looking foolish."

Time, like a snowflake, disappears while we are trying to
decide what to do with it.

ST. LOUIS BUGLE

Tamara is on an emotional high when she describes this particular group on the phone to me. "Jeez, Maryann, this group was one of
my best. They're moving. They're changing," she says.

I've been living with the letters, but she has been immersed with
the real people. I can just picture her. After hanging up, I turn on the
computer, open a new file, and start writing . . . not our joint answers
to the letter writers who have made me want to cry, but a book.
Tamara's letter writers will wait, I hope. Perhaps a book will be inspiration enough to help them start their journeys.

We are, first, human beings. And so when you weep, I
understand it clearly. When you laugh, I understand it clearly.
When you love, you don't have to translate it to me. These are
the important things.

MAYA ANGELOU, WOMAN AS WRITER

Tamara's Journey . . . in Her Own Words

At the Dunkin' Donuts in Upper Montclair:

In the fall of 1995, I applied for a job as a fitness instructor at Aiken
Regional Medical Centers over in Aiken, South Carolina. Someone I
knew from a health club in Augusta had been working there and recommended that I go for it. I had been doing all my work, all my teaching, right there on Fort Gordon, and moving out and away like this,
if only for part of my time, was really exciting.

I wanted to teach classes at the hospital on Monday, Wednesday,
and Friday evenings from 5:30 to 6:30 and be one of their regular fitness instructors. It was so exciting for me, even though I knew that it
would mean a bit of a hardship for my kids. But I could still be there
when they arrived home from school and head on over to Aiken, a
forty-five-minute drive, after everyone was settled and doing home-

work. I was hired. Shoot, it was wonderful, and I felt as if I was on my way. There would be no stopping me now.

I began to think of not only fitness as a career option for me but also becoming a motivational speaker. My students liked the light-hearted, do-whatever-you-can approach I had to exercise. They also loved the idea that I had been a really fat gal. Through Aiken Regional, I used to be asked to speak to various corporations and community groups. The University of South Carolina, the Aiken Mall, the Wey-erhaeuser Corporation, Aiken Technical College, and the Newcomers' Club all loved my presentations. The next thing I knew, my classes expanded to five days a week.

About that same time, I went on the early morning local news doing fitness spots and then again at night sometimes. People were see-ing this woman, me, and saying, "What is she trying to say?" Viewers were catching bits and pieces of my "Love Self, Think Health, Move It to Lose It" message and asking questions. Where could they find Fat Chat? Shoot! This face and this voice were really out there in the public eye, and I realized that I could be doing more for my commu-nity than simply teaching exercise and good nutrition. I had lost all that weight and become healthy. Everyone wanted to know how. Other support groups at the hospital existed, so I went to my superiors with the idea of a group that would meet weekly to share stories and express how much we cared about each other.

Reaching your optimal body composition and creating health through food choices happens in your mind and body simultaneously.

CHRISTINE NORTHRUP, M.D.,
WOMEN'S BODIES, WOMEN'S WISDOM

My very first Fat Chat sessions started in April 1996. We met on Wednesdays, after aerobics classes, from 6:45 to 7:45 P.M., right there in the Aurora Pavilion gym. Five or six people showed up, having seen the notice of it in the hospital's *Quality of Life* magazine which is dis-tributed free of charge, four times a year, to the community, publi-cizing the variety of support groups, educational programs, and seminars at the hospital. I would have considered it a success if only one person attended.

The support group was my way of putting my own experience right out there to see if I could help others. I told the group that first evening that we were just going to get together to chat and share. Everyone kind of laughed about sharing and caring with no rules—my idea hit home right away. We weren't going to do what I called "Mickey-Mouse" around the topic of fat, either. We were all going to be open. In fact, in the beginning, I wasn't as much of an instructor as I was a participant. Now I've got more of a message to get across or certain points I try to make. Even so, sometimes, no matter what week we are in, I'll sit down and say, "Awwww heck, let's just talk."

Meanwhile, the strength I was finding in dealing with my health, promoting my ideas in the professional world, and staying committed to my journey helped me decide that I didn't need to take the abuse at home from my ex-husband quietly. When he scared me and frightened the children to death, I had the military police step into our lives. It took almost a year to get the authorities to believe that I was battered. Finally, he was sentenced to nine months of confinement. We were divorced in March 1997. That time was a trip to hell and back, but I refused to give up my quest to stay healthy.

Mine is the only program I know that offers sound advice along with counseling, discussion, and support. Participants are never judged by those three numbers on the scale, but by the health and lifestyle changes they are able to make. I also produced a video demo and a press kit, and with the help of my poppa and my oldest brother, Ed, I incorporated my business. It's been going strong ever since. I'll never slide back. I'm a role model for my kids, my Fat Chat gals, and people everywhere. I'm tellin' you the truth: If I can change my life, you can too. You can rewrite your own story.

This is my way . . .
What is your way?
The *way doesn't exist.*

Friedrich Nietzsche

9

"Now It's Your Turn"
To Lose 100 Pounds . . .

Imagination is the beginning of creation. You imagine what you desire; you will what you imagine; and at last you create what you will.

GEORGE BERNARD SHAW

My Third-Floor Office, Montclair, New Jersey:

Watching the women in Fat Chat with Tamara groups put together new patterns of living, I've noticed that each seems to pick and choose from a varied menu of options. They get excited about walking, about doing a step aerobics class without using the step, about finding fat-free foods to love as well as meal planning for energy, and about understanding and moving their bodies in new ways. Linda isn't taking the same route that Ann has adopted. Monique and Peggy are in another camp. Someone else is going swimming three nights a week in the Aurora pool. And a crew of regulars wouldn't miss Tamara's nightly aerobic workouts for the world.

You have your own path to choose. As Tamara has said to me over and over again, it begins with the three basic principles: "Love Self!

Think Health! Move It to Lose It!"After that, your journey can be one that is virtually incomparable to anyone else's . . . even people to whom you pass along this very book.

When I look behind at the logic of Tamara's program, a somewhat strange image comes to my mind: a Chinese restaurant take-out menu with hundreds of delicious and good-for-you suggestions to try. No matter what you choose, you will end up satisfied. In designing your own personal program, the important thing is to make your selections and to take some from column A (New Healthier Habits) along with some from column B (Exercise) and column C (Love Yourself), too.

At Aiken Regional Medical Centers where the program first developed, the self-help sessions were set up using a sixteen-week format, but only because the hospital's *Quality of Life* magazine is distributed four times a year. This publication promotes all the wellness programs offered at the medical centers. Every four months was a time frame that suited the publishing schedule . . . nothing more and nothing magical about this timing. "I don't care if you spend sixteen weeks, sixteen days, or sixteen minutes," Tamara says.

She encourages everyone to take advantage of the knowledge to be gained, pointing out that since its inception, Fat Chat has become more content-specific. "When I first began holding the sessions, I didn't have very much of my program down on paper. After about a year of just hanging out, sharing, caring, and chatting in that semicircle of chairs, I began to see the value of the instructional side of the process. Yes, you need to be inspired, but you also need information. Meanwhile, I had picked up so much information that I wanted to share. Sometimes we even meet in a conference room where I have this big marking board to use."

Here are brief descriptions of what often happens in the sixteen sessions of Fat Chat with Tamara. Feel free to skip around, and be sure to include some of the suggestions from the "Right Now, Do It Today" listing at the end of this section. Choose some from Move It to Lose It, some from Think Health, and some from Love Self.

Session One In the first session, "I introduce myself, offer an overview of the program, and ask participants if they have questions, and then they register," Tamara explains. That initial registration includes basic medical information. In fact, before you begin to design your own program, you'll want to speak with your health-care provider. If you have not been physically active and have any preexisting health condition, scheduling a checkup is a must. Take this book with you to show your health practitioner.

In class, Tamara asks participants:

What is the present state of your general health?

Are you currently taking medications?

Does your physician know you are participating in this program?

What regular physical activity are you doing now?

The key idea introduced on that first night together is: Put your scale out of sight and temporarily out of mind. Stop weighing yourself. Hide the scale under the clothes hamper if you must.

> *Take a chance. All life is a chance. The man who goes farthest is generally the one who is willing to do and dare.*
>
> DALE CARNEGIE'S SCRAPBOOK

If time permits, Fat Chat participants begin to examine their behavioral patterns by taking a quiz. Working with Sandy Hobbs, a registered nurse and the former director of marketing at Aiken Regional Medical Centers, Tamara developed the questionnaire to help people become more aware of their behaviors. Sometimes the quiz-taking spills over to the second meeting. Or, people may choose to take the form home so they can spend quiet, uninterrupted time thinking about themselves.

You can do it here. Pull out a pencil, sit down, take this quiz:

Keep in mind that there are no right or wrong answers. You don't have to share your results with a living soul, so you can be honest. Remember, you are accountable to you and only you. Some of the questions may seem repetitive, silly, or intrusive, but the idea is to bring you to a turning point. Sometimes as we all race through busy lives, it's difficult to remember where we've been emotionally and physically as well as where we are heading. So, find a quiet spot where you won't be interrupted, and take your time.

1. As a child, you were:

   - underweight
   - ideal weight
   - somewhat overweight
   - very overweight

2. Do you remember when you first became aware that you had a weight problem? How old were you?

3. When you were growing up, did you expect to be _____ as an adult?

   - underweight
   - ideal weight
   - somewhat overweight
   - very overweight

We are what we repeatedly do. Excellence, then, is not an act, but a habit.

ARISTOTLE

4. Your father was _____ when you were a child.

   - underweight
   - ideal weight
   - somewhat overweight
   - very overweight

5. Your mother was _____ when you were a child.

   - underweight
   - ideal weight
   - somewhat overweight
   - very overweight

6. Was food used to make you feel better and heal your hurts when you were a child?

   - never
   - rarely

- frequently
- usually

A dream is what you would like for life to be and hold, but a goal is what you intend to make happen.

DENNIS WAITLEY

7. Were you physically active as a child?

- not at all
- slightly
- somewhat
- highly

8. How often do you weigh yourself?

- daily
- 2–5 times a week
- weekly
- monthly
- less than once a month

9. Are you concerned about your weight and eating behavior?

- not at all
- slightly
- a great deal
- tremendously

Fitness experts used to be impatient with people who just couldn't get moving. These days, most of us in this profession are more realistic. We recognize that it's hard to translate knowledge into action, and we're learning more and more about how to help.

MIRIAM NELSON, PH.D., *STRONG WOMEN STAY YOUNG*

10. Do you see overeating and being overweight as your biggest problem?

- yes
- no

11. How often do you think about your weight?

- almost never
- occasionally
- frequently
- almost daily
- daily

12. Are you feeling guilty about being fat?

- not at all
- slightly
- quite a bit
- extremely

13. Do you like and enjoy your body?

- not at all
- just a little
- quite a bit
- a lot

14. Do you look at yourself in a full-length mirror without wearing any clothes?

- never
- rarely
- frequently
- daily

No matter how far you have gone on a wrong road, turn back.

TURKISH PROVERB

15. How often do you feel full?

- never
- rarely
- frequently
- daily
- more than once a day

16. How often are you aware of your body's signals of fullness?

    - never
    - rarely
    - frequently
    - daily
    - more than once a day

17. Physically speaking, where do you feel comfortably full?

    - at my waistline
    - a few inches above the waistline
    - at breast level
    - in my throat

18. Do you eat in response to either stress, loneliness, anger, boredom, or anxiety?

    - never
    - rarely
    - frequently
    - daily

19. Are you preoccupied with food and eating?
    - never
    - sometimes
    - frequently

20. How many foods are you powerless to resist or avoid overeating?

    - none
    - 1–3
    - 4–6
    - more than 6

21. Do you feel guilty when you eat these danger foods?

    - yes
    - no

22. If you were to rate eating as a form of recreation in your life, how would you describe it?

    - unimportant
    - slightly important

- rather important
- very important

23. How many eating or drinking pals can you count?

  - none
  - 1–2
  - 3–4
  - 5–6
  - more than 6

24. How often do you reward yourself with food?

  - never
  - rarely
  - frequently
  - regularly

25. Do you use food to show your affection toward other people?

  - never
  - sometimes
  - frequently
  - regularly

26. Would you prefer that other people not see what, how much, or how often you eat?

  - yes
  - no

Since habits become power, make them work with you and not against you.

E. Stanley Jones

27. How often do you consider yourself powerless to resist the urge to eat even when you aren't hungry?

  - never
  - occasionally
  - frequently
  - usually

28. Can you resist food when it's being offered?

    - never
    - rarely
    - frequently
    - regularly

29. How often do you eat fast foods in a week?

    - never
    - 1–3 times
    - 4–6 times
    - more than 6 times

30. How often do you eat in your car?

    - never
    - rarely
    - frequently
    - regularly

Since it takes twenty minutes for the appetite center in the brain to register satiety, eating too fast is likely to result in overeating.

VICTOR HERBERT, M.D., *THE MOUNT SINAI SCHOOL OF MEDICINE COMPLETE BOOK OF NUTRITION*

31. Do you hide food or eat secretly?

    - yes
    - no
    - occasionally

32. Do food ads make you want to eat even when you aren't really hungry?

    - yes
    - no
    - occasionally

33. How often do you binge or overeat?

- never
- rarely
- frequently
- regularly

34. How many times a day do you eat?

35. How would you describe the pace of your meals?

    - slow
    - somewhat slow
    - quick
    - faster than anyone else at the table

36. Would you describe your food choices as nutritious?

    - never
    - rarely
    - frequently

37. How often do you discover that you've gobbled down food so fast that you haven't really tasted it?

    - never
    - rarely
    - frequently

38. How often do you crave sweets?

    - never
    - rarely
    - frequently

39. How often do you feel tired or lethargic during the day?

    - never
    - rarely
    - frequently

40. Do you have trouble sleeping?

    - yes
    - no

41. How often do you exercise?

- never
- rarely
- once a week
- 2–3 times a week
- more than 3 times a week

42. Do you like exercising?

43. Think about it. What would make you exercise more often?

- free time
- convenience
- motivation
- something else? _____

New research indicates that your exercise habits have as much to say about your size as your genes do.

HEALTH MAGAZINE

44. Do you know how to exercise without getting hurt?

45. Do you understand the benefits of regular exercise?

46. Count up all the diets you've ever been on.

47. Can you remember the average length of time you stuck to any of these reducing plans?

48. What do you like most about being on a diet?

49. What do you like least about being on a diet?

50. How would you characterize your commitment to becoming healthier now?

- low
- medium
- high

51. Take a wild guess at the name of the person who will ultimately make it possible for you to lose weight this time, once and for all. (If you said Tamara Hill, you are not quite at your turning point—yet.)

Session Two Session two of Fat Chat continues the exploration into self-awareness. Tamara will ask, "Are you ready? Where are you right now?" Sometimes, more time is devoted to the fifty-one questions from the previous session. "Knowledge about yourself is so powerful," Tamara tells participants.

Another survey is handed out which asks, "Over the course of your life, approximately how much weight have you lost? Approximately how much of the weight that you lost was eventually regained? Women— and yes, they are mostly women—consider five reasons they want to lose weight.

Take some time to write down the five principal reasons why you want to lose weight. Don't promise yourself that you'll make your list later. Do it now. In fact, find an empty notebook or folder, and label it "Fat Chat." In classes, participants receive a glossy folder with purple and blue lettering and a cover design that states: "Fat Chat . . . changing lives for the better." Consider making your own to store the book, results of your quiz, as well as surveys, tips, ideas, and inspirational quotations.

Session Three In session number three, Tamara usually focuses on goal setting and asks participants to brainstorm and find their long-term, short-range, and ninety-day as well as daily goals. "Where do you want to end up?" she asks. The operative idea on this night is that "Your dreams belong to you and only you," she explains.

As she herself learned on her own journey, you can't be accountable to a scale, a chart, your mate, the doctor, or anyone but yourself if you are to succeed. Participants are also asked to list the rewards they will give themselves for achieving each goal. This may be fun. "Spend at least five minutes a day visualizing yourself making progress toward your goals," she suggests. Build this into your everyday life, because it's easy and uplifting. For instance, before you go to sleep at night, focus on those goals. Or find another time of day to spend on yourself and your goals.

Perfection is an unrealistic destination. . . . There is no state of perfection on the map, and if you continually go looking for it, you may miss the really good stuff . . . and spoil your trip. Relax and enjoy the ride.

KAY WILLIS, *Are We Having Fun Yet?*
The 16 Secrets of Happy Parenting

Session Four Chat sessions don't always run rigidly on schedule, nor do they exclude any issue someone wants to raise. In fact, food and exercise are always above and beneath the buzz of the official topic of conversation. In session four, Tamara tries to return to the issue of self-acceptance. "Who are you?" she asks. "Do you like yourself? If not, why not? Accept yourself. Stop thinking that you need to be punished. You don't have to settle for where you are, but in order to change your lifestyle, you must work on your mind first. The brain is the center of everything, so you need to feed your head positive thoughts.

"Understand this," she tells participants, "too many weight-loss programs equate success with loss. Their standard of success is built only on your loss of pounds and not on your gaining knowledge and new habits. Eating as well as exercising become unnatural or unnaturally difficult and rooted in feeling bad about yourself."

Make a list of your habits, both good and bad. Let's take examples of good first:

- You walk instead of driving as much as possible.
- You bike to that bakery.
- You weight-train two to three times a week.
- You are stretching or doing flexibility exercises regularly.
- You eat low-fat foods most of the time.
- You eat breakfast every morning.
- You eat at least three to five small meals per day.
- You drink alcohol only in moderation.
- You don't smoke.
- You have your blood pressure, blood cholesterol level, and blood sugar checked every six months.
- You make a conscious effort to avoid salt.
- You always wear your seat belt when you are in a car.
- Add your own.

Now, take a look at some examples of bad habits:

- You don't always get six to eight hours of sleep.
- You don't drink eight to ten glasses of water a day.
- You use food as an emotional comfort when you are stressed out.
- You don't eat as many fruits or vegetables as you should. (Five servings of each is the amount recommended by dietitians.)
- You don't reward yourself for your achievements.

- You don't take twenty minutes or more to eat a meal.
- You don't eat at least two healthy, low-fat snacks a day.
- Add your own.

Session Five For session number five, if she has a blackboard handy, Tamara will write: "Changes, Choices, Challenges," and then lead the discussion into how to "face change positively." Each participant considers her own formula for change, and solutions for overcoming obstacles are shared. "Most people make statements like, 'Well, fat is in my family, and there's nothing I can do about my weight,'" Tamara explains. "They say, 'It's hereditary. It's genetic.' That's bull. You still have choices.

"Every choice you make—chocolate versus white cake, a high-fat candy bar versus a bag of fat-free Starbursts, a sugary soda versus a bottle of water—every choice you make has a consequence. The point is, that choice is up to you," Tamara says.

Most people, though not everyone, decide to keep a daily food diary, at least for several days. Try it. You might find it beneficial. Buy a small, pocketbook-size notebook and keep it handy so you can jot down what you are eating during the day. You don't have to continue keeping your food diary for weeks or months on end and some people hate making lists. However, Tamara notes that a little record keeping helps to make you aware of eating habits.

Plain water . . . at least eight glasses a day . . . is actually a wonderful aid to weight loss. It aids the kidneys in flushing impurities out of the system, reducing the dehydration that causes skin to appear dry and lined.

CHERYL HARTSOUGH, *THE ANTI-CELLULITE DIET*

Session Six In session number six, Tamara dives into one of her favorite topics: "Dieting—Truly a Losing Game." The chatting centers on why diets don't work and what's wrong with all the short-term, quick-fix remedies. Her key idea is that you are being prompted to try bizarre and dangerous diets every day of your life. "You starve yourself. You go to fat farms. You take harmful drugs. You spend far too much money at weight-loss clinics," she says. "You may even have lost

Basic Nutrition

Establishing healthier food habits can help you reduce your risk of high blood cholesterol. By reducing your risk of high blood cholesterol, you reduce your risk for heart attacks. By eating less fat, especially saturated (animal) fats, you will keep your cholesterol level down and also control your weight.

Following is a practical guide to the basic food groups, with the number of servings per day recommended by the American Heart Association. Choose a variety of foods from each group. (These guidelines differ slightly from the portions recommended in the Food Guide Pyramid on page 124, but the underlying aim is similiar.)

Breads, cereals, pasta, and starchy vegetables (6 servings per day)

1 serving equals:
1 slice bread
$1/2$ cup cereal, rice, pasta
$1/4$ to $1/2$ cup starchy vegatables (corn or potatoes)

Vegetables and fruits (5 or more servings per day)

1 serving equals:
a medium-size piece of fruit
$1/2$ cup fruit juice
$1/2$ to 1 cup cooked or raw vegetables
Olives and avocados count as fats.

Meat, poultry, and fish (no more than 6 cooked ounces per day)

1 serving equals:
3-ounce portion (about the size of a deck of cards) meat
$1/2$ chicken breast
$3/4$ cup flaked fish
1 cup cooked beans, peas, or lentils
3 ounces tofu
Trim fat from meats; remove skin from poultry.

Dairy products (2 to 4 servings per day)

1 serving equals:
1 cup low-fat milk or yogurt (2% milk is not low-fat)
1 ounce cheese (no more than 3 grams of fat per ounce)

Eggs (no more than 3 to 4 egg yolks a week)

Egg whites aren't limited, because they don't contain cholesterol.

Fats and oils (no more than 5 to 8 servings per day)

1 serving equals:
1 teaspoon vegetable oil or regular margarine
2 teaspoons diet margarine
1 tablespoon salad dressing
2 teaspoons mayonnaise or peanut butter
1 tablespoon seed or nuts
$1/8$ medium avocado
10 small or 5 large olives

weight—for a while," she adds. However, only 3 to 5 percent of people who lose weight on restrictive diets manage to keep it off." (See Basic Nutrition on page 123.)

Session Seven Eating behavior is up for discussion in session number seven. "Where do you eat? Do you plan meals? What triggers you to eat? Can you recognize the basic food groups? Are you choosing dairy products, the right kind of fats, carbohydrates, proteins? Do you eat from every group on the food guide pyramid?

"Let's talk about replacing negative habits with positive ones," she will ask the group. The lesson to be learned is that there is no evil food. "I've lost 100 pounds, and I've kept it off. Yet, I eat anything I want to eat," she informs the class. Mental health must be part of your plan: "A piece of paper with a list of bad foods, especially if that list includes things you love, will drive you crazy sooner or later and probably sooner."

Food Guide Pyramid
A Guide to Daily Food Choices

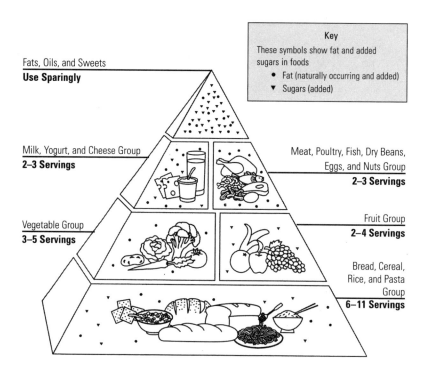

Key
These symbols show fat and added sugars in foods
• Fat (naturally occurring and added)
▼ Sugars (added)

Fats, Oils, and Sweets
Use Sparingly

Milk, Yogurt, and Cheese Group
2–3 Servings

Meat, Poultry, Fish, Dry Beans, Eggs, and Nuts Group
2–3 Servings

Vegetable Group
3–5 Servings

Fruit Group
2–4 Servings

Bread, Cereal, Rice, and Pasta Group
6–11 Servings

If one advances confidently in the direction of his dreams, and endeavors to live the life which he has imagined, he will meet with a success unexpected in common hours. If you have built castles in the air, your work need not be lost, that is where they should be. Now put the foundations under them.

THOREAU

Session Eight In session number eight, food and learning how to eat healthier still lead the discussion list. Learn some facts about foods. You don't need to become a fanatic or go for a Ph.D in nutrition science. A basic understanding is going to take you a long way toward your goal. Participants bring in nutrition labels, and Tamara takes them mentally down their favorite grocery store aisles so the discussion can center on calories, serving sizes, fats, and other important nutritional concepts. (See How to Read a Nutrition Label on page 126.)

Making modifications in your diet is not as difficult as you may now imagine. "The real trick is to make small, seriously just tiny, changes in your eating habits every day," Tamara explains. To help, the following table of high-fat versus low-fat preparation methods is offered:

More recipe preparation tips are exchanged, and Tamara's take-home handout includes these suggestions:

- If a recipe calls for whole milk or cream, use skim, or canned, evaporated skim, or low-fat milk instead.
- If the recipe calls for sour cream, substitute plain yogurt. In food that is to be heated, mix in 1 tablespoon of flour for each cup of yogurt to prevent separation.
- If the recipe or meal calls for high-fat cheese, use half the amount or find a substitute cheese with a lower fat content.
- If the recipe calls for mayonnaise, use half the amount or less, or substitute fat-free yogurt.
- If the recipe calls for baking chocolate, use three tablespoons of cocoa powder plus one tablespoon of vegetable oil for each ounce recommended.

For times when you crave fast food, Tamara offers a list of new possibilities. Instead of your old regular, fatty treats . . .

How to Read a Nutrition Label

Serving Size

Is your serving size the same as the one on the label? If you eat double the serving size listed, you need to double the nutrient and calorie values. If you eat one-half the serving size shown here, cut the nutrient and calorie values in half.

Calories

Are you overweight? Cut back a little on calories! Look here to see how a serving of the food adds to your daily total.

Total Carbohydrate

When you cut down on fat, you can have more carbohydrates. Carbohydrates are in foods such as bread, potatoes, fruits, and vegetables. Choose these often!

Dietary Fiber

Grandmother called it "roughage," but her advice to eat more is still up to date! That goes for both soluble and insoluble kinds of dietary fiber. Fruits, vegetables, whole-grain foods, beans, and peas are all good sources and can help reduce the risk of heart disease and cancer.

Protein

Most Americans get more protein than they need. Where there is animal protein, there is also fat and cholesterol.

Vitamins and Minerals

Your goal here is 100% of each for the day. Don't count on one food to do it all. Let a combination of foods add up to a winning score.

Total Fat

Aim low. Most people need to cut back on fat! Too much fat may contribute to heart disease and cancer. Try to limit your calories from fat.

Saturated Fat

A new kind of fat? No, saturated fat is part of the total fat in foods. It is listed separately because it's the key player in raising blood cholesterol and your risk of heart disease. Eat less!

Cholesterol

Too much cholesterol, a second cousin to fat, can lead to heart disease. Challenge yourself to eat less than 300 g each day.

Sodium

You call it "salt"; the label calls it "sodium." Either way, it may add up to high blood pressure

---

Nutrition Facts

Serving Size 2 pieces (32 grams)
Servings per Container 12

Amount per Serving	
Calories 130	Calories from fat 10

%Daily Value*

Total Fat 1g	1%
Saturated Fat 0g	0%
Polyunsaturated Fat 0g	0%
Monounsaturated Fat 0g	0%
Cholesterol 0mg	0%
Sodium 40mg	2%
Potassium 50mg	2%
Total Carbohydrate 25g	8%
Dietary Fiber 1g	4%
Sugars 1g	
Protein 3g	

Vitamin A 0%		Vitamin C	0%
Calcium 0%		Iron	8%

*Percent Daily Values are based on a 2,000 calorie diet. Your daily values may be higher or lower depending on your calorie needs.

	Calories:	2,000	2,500
Total Fat	Less than	65g	80g
Saturated Fat	Less than	20g	25g
Cholesterol	Less than	300g	300mg
Sodium	Less than	2,400mg	2,400mg
Total Carbohydrates		300g	375g
Dietary Fiber		25g	30g

Calories per gram:

Fat 9 • Carbohydrate 4 • Protein 4

---

in some people. So, keep your sodium intake low, 2,400 to 3,000 mg or less each day.

Daily Value

Feel as if you're drowning in numbers? Let the Daily Value be your guide. Daily Values are listed for people who eat 2,000 or 2,500 calories each day.

g = grams (About 28g = 1 ounce) mg = milligrams (1,000 mg = 1g)

High Fat	Lower Fat
Pan-fry	Bake
Deep-fat fry	Stir-fry; broil (use rack so fat drips off); poach; steam; microwave; roast (use rack so fat drips off)
Sauté in butter, margarine, or oil	Cut fat by sautéing in broth or wine; use nonstick pans or cooking spray
Baste meats with pan drippings	Baste with wine, broth, or vegetable or fruit juices
Pan-cook ground meat	Cook well, drain fat, rinse in colander
Use lard, bacon grease, or chicken fat	Omit or use half the amount, rely on herbs to flavor
Fat in homemade soups and stews	Cook a day ahead so you can chill and remove hardened fat from the surface, then reheat and serve

At McDonald's, order:

- McGrilled Chicken Classic, or
- Chunky Chicken Salad, or
- Side salad with diet dressing, or
- Garden salad with diet dressing

At Taco Bell, order:

- Lite Chicken Tacos, or
- Lite Taco Supreme, or
- Lite Tacos, or
- Lite Soft Tacos

At Arby's, order:

- Light Roast Chicken Deluxe, or
- Light Roast Turkey Deluxe, or

- Plain Baked Potato, or
- Side salad with diet dressing

At Wendy's, order:

- Grilled Chicken Filet, or
- Chili with crackers, or
- Baked Potato, or
- Garden salad with diet dressing

At Hardee's, order:

- Regular Roast Beef, or
- Grilled Chicken Sandwich, or
- Side salad with diet dressing

What's great all year? Bananas, carrots, celery, coconuts, eggplant, garlic, ginger, herbs, kiwis, lemons, limes, melons, mushrooms, onions, parsley, snow peas, pineapples, potatoes, radishes, scallions, sprouts, watercress.

Session Nine In session number nine, Tamara discusses how to chart your progress. While there is never any rigid weigh-in ritual, twice in the original sixteen-week program, participants get on a scale standing backward so that pounds can be recorded but they can't see the actual number. Chest, waist, hips, biceps, thighs, and calf measurements are also taken and recorded. If you decide to work with your doctor creating this individualized plan, you may also be able to use your blood sugar levels, blood pressure readings, and cholesterol count as measures of progress.(See Individual Data Record on page 129.)

"Every day, treat yourself in some small way," she tells them this week as well as in many others. Rewards are a consistent theme. You can do this for yourself at home. "Think about what would make you really happy today, and then go for it," Tamara coaches.

Other ways of measuring progress are discussed, including body mass index (BMI), waist-to-hip ratio (WHR), and the skinfold calipers test.

Individual Data Record

Initial Measurements

Chest	____	Biceps	____
Waist	____	Thigh	____
Hips	____	Calf	____

Date	Weight	Lbs. Lost	Total Lbs. Lost	Total Inches Lost	Blood Sugar	Blood Pressure	Cholesterol

Your Ideal Weight

The guidelines apply to adult men and women alike, regardless of age.

Height	Healthy Weight	Moderately Overweight	Severely Overweight
4'10"	92–120 lbs.	121–140 lbs.	141–250 lbs.
4'11"	95–125 lbs.	126–145 lbs.	146–250 lbs.
5'	98–128 lbs.	129–150 lbs.	151–250 lbs.
5'1"	101–132 lbs.	133–152 lbs.	153–250 lbs.
5'2"	105–138 lbs.	139–158 lbs.	159–250 lbs.
5'3"	109–140 lbs.	141–163 lbs.	164–250 lbs.
5'4"	112–148 lbs.	149–170 lbs.	171–250 lbs.
5'5"	115–150 lbs.	151–175 lbs.	176–250 lbs.
5'6"	119–155 lbs.	156–180 lbs.	181–250 lbs.
5'7"	122–160 lbs.	161–185 lbs.	186–250 lbs.
5'8"	126–163 lbs.	164–190 lbs.	191–250 lbs.
5'9"	130–170 lbs.	171–196 lbs.	197–250 lbs.
5'10"	133–173 lbs.	174–203 lbs.	204–250 lbs.
5'11"	138–178 lbs.	179–208 lbs.	209–250 lbs.
6'	141–185 lbs.	186–215 lbs.	216–250 lbs.
6'1"	145–190 lbs.	191–220 lbs.	221–250 lbs.
6'2"	148–195 lbs.	196–225 lbs.	226–250 lbs.

Weighing Beyond the Scale

Three ways to measure your body's fat:

Body Mass Index (BMI)

The use of Quetelet's index, or body mass index (BMI), is a unique expression of height-to-weight and is more closely related to body fatness, as determined through hydrostatic weighing, than are standardized height/weight tables. From this measure, a high BMI is positively associated with hypertension, high blood cholesterol levels, and cardiorespiratory disease. A healthy BMI is about 20–25.

Waist-to-Hip Ratio (WHR)

One means of addressing regional fat distribution if you are overweight is to assess and compare circumferences of the waist and hip, referred to as the waist-to-hip ratio (WHR). To determine this ratio, the accurate measurement of both waist and hip circumferences is essential. Divide your waist size by your hip size, and you get a key to how much fat is stored in the abdomen. The lowest healthy ratio is not yet known. Many experts agree that women with ratios of .8 or lower and men with ratios of 1 or lower are in good shape.

Skinfold Calipers (Pinch Test)

Special calipers are used to measure folds of skin and fat in several spots on the body and average them. It is not a precise method; a reading of 25 percent body fat could mean an actual number as high as 28 or as low as 22—or could be even further off with a badly trained technician.

> *Fun is not frivolous; it is essential, play is imperative. Playfulness is the door to surprise, possibility, invention, and breakthroughs."*
>
> JOLINE GODFREY, *OUR WILDEST DREAMS*

Session Ten While moving a little more every day has been part of the process, in week number ten, Tamara gives extra attention to exercise. She distributes a cautionary handout which states: "Before beginning any exercise program, check with your doctor first." Take her advice as you start this journey at home on your own.

For most people, physical activity should not pose any problem or harm, and no medical clearance is ordinarily needed. Exercise does not have to hurt to be good for you. Schedule time for exercise in your appointment book or on your calendar. What kind of exercise do you like best: fun? a formal program? everyday movement that is functionally a part of your life? family outings? Exercise does not have to be a frightening word that makes you cringe in embarrassment or exhaustion before you even begin. Think baby steps here.

"Listen to your body. It knows best. Remember to start off slowly and progress gradually. You'll get there, don't worry," she says. "I'm not talking about signing up at a health club populated with stick-thin twenty-year-olds proud to be hopping around in their spare-no-embarrassment spandex," Tamara insists. "All I want you to do is get up and move your body. Today. A little more tomorrow. And a little more every day. I know you can find something that you love to do."

"The health benefits associated with regular exercise are phenomenal," Tamara states. Exercise . . .

- Reduces the risk of cardiovascular disease:

    - Increases HDL (good) cholesterol—levels of less than 35 mg/dl (milligrams per deciliter) are considered low
    - Decreases LDL (bad) cholesterol—levels of 130 mg/dl and below are ideal
    - Decreases triglyceride levels—levels above 250 mg/dl are considered high
    - Promotes relaxation; relieves stress, tension, anxiety, and depression
    - Decreases body fat and favorably changes body composition
    - Increases energy level and metabolism
    - Reduces blood pressure, especially if it is high

- Helps control diabetes:

    - Makes cells less resistant to insulin
    - Reduces body fat

- Develops stronger bones that are less susceptible to injury
- Contributes to fewer low-back problems
- Acts as a stimulus for other lifestyle changes
- Improves self-image and self-esteem
- Helps decrease rate and impact of aging (reduced mortality)

Participants soon learn:

- A *warm-up* gradually increases heart rate and body temperature and helps ensure that joints and muscles are ready for activity.
- A *cool down* allows slow, gradual recovery of your normal heart rate after an aerobic workout and prevents pooling of blood in your lower extremities.

Though handouts may stress technical points in an exercise program, or offer a formula for calculating your target heart-rate zone during an aerobic workout, the really good news for you is that you can be excused from the technicalities. *Anything* you do is well worth your effort. "Put down the remote control," Tamara says. "Take the stairs instead of the elevator."

Session Eleven Exercise is still on the agenda in session eleven. "Please, puhleeesseee . . . keep at it." Sometimes, the talk turns to exercise machines, but more often than not, the chat will include ideas for remaining more flexible, for gaining strength, and for tightening the abdominal muscles.

"No amount of crunches or torso twists will get rid of excess fat around your midsection. On the other hand, regular aerobic exercise and a diet low in fat will," Tamara explains. "Not everyone can achieve a chiseled midsection, but it is possible to develop strong abdominal muscles, thereby strengthening the back. Abdominal strength and endurance play an important role in the prevention of low-back pain. Likewise, more important than looking better, losing fat around your midsection will help you maintain a healthy heart."

She emphasizes proper technique to maximize results as well as avoid injury. "A very important thing to remember when you are exercising your abdominal muscles is to use correct form," she teaches. Before you get down on your bedroom floor to try a sit-up (or what she calls the "basic crunch"), remember:

- Don't pull on your neck. Keep your chin off your chest.
- Don't throw your body, or use jerking motions to complete the exercise. Keep your abdominal muscles pulled in tight, with your back flat against your mat.
- Always exhale as you contract your abdominal muscles while lifting your chest. Inhale as you release and lower your chest back down to your mat.

According to Tamara, the "basic crunch" is the best abdominal exercise to tone and strengthen the upper abdominals. This exercise is performed with your knees bent and your back flat on your mat. Raise your chest and shoulders off the mat, exhaling as you come up and inhaling as you go back down.

To work the muscles on the sides of your midsection, perform this basic crunch at alternating angles, reaching with your shoulder (not your elbow) across the body to the opposite knee. Now do the same thing on your other side.

To work the muscles in the lower abdominal area, bring your knees up toward your chest, forming a ninety-degree angle with your body. Using only your lower abdominals and not your legs or hips, bring your knees slightly toward your chest as you exhale. Return to the starting position. This is a very small movement, so don't try to bring your knees up to your face.

There are no set rules about the number of repetitions. Beginners may be able to do one set of four to eight repetitions. If you can do only one, do it. "Remember, if I can do it, so can you, and I had to crawl, practically, before I could walk and then run," Tamara says. As you train your abdominals, you will be able to work up to three sets of eight to twelve repetitions.

Weight resistance is also a hot topic in exercise chat sessions. "Strength training, or working with weights, has been said to be one of the best activities to help prevent aging. The primary reason," Tamara explains, "is that weight resistance training increases muscle mass, which increases the caloric needs of the additional lean muscle mass. In turn, your body's metabolism (the rate at which you burn calories) increases." Working with weights will

- Increase the strength of your bones, muscles, and connective tissue, decreasing your risk of injury.
- Increase your muscle mass. (Did you know that the average adult loses about one-half pound of lean muscle per year after age twenty?)
- Enhance your quality of life. (As your strength increases, the effort required to perform your daily tasks will be less taxing.)

Investigate weight-training programs near your home. Working with an experienced trainer may be important for beginners. A book such as *Strong Women Stay Young* by Miriam E. Nelson, Ph.D., can also help you get started. The important thing is to take the first step.

Session Twelve The idea presented in session twelve is that you must accentuate the positive parts of your body. "The average American woman is 5′4″ tall and weighs 142 pounds. The average model on the cover of a magazine or on your television screen weighs 110 pounds and is 5′10″ tall. I'm pretty sure that you can't become that 'perfect' model without paying a high price. For God's sake, stop beating yourself up mentally and think health, not looks," Tamara insists. Participants receive a handout describing body types which includes definitions of *mesomorph*, *ectomorph*, and *endomorph*. Which type best describes you?

• **Are you a mesomorph?** Strong, athletic, you build muscle easily. You look athletic, and in fact, you are. Of all the body types, you're the best at sports. You have muscular shoulders that are wider than your hips. Your muscles get bigger as they get stronger. As a mesomorph, you risk looking overweight when you're really just solid. Mesomorphs usually have 22 to 28 percent body fat, and extra fat tends to end up in the midsection.

What's best for mesomorphs? Mesomorphs need to do thirty to forty-five minutes of aerobic exercise four to six times a week. Weight training with medium resistance, high repetitions; jumping rope; bicycling in slow gears for lower resistance; distance running; modern dance; and ballet are just a few of the best body-enhancing sports for this body type.

• **Are you an ectomorph?** Sleek, angular, you can get toned quickly. Your shoulders and hips are about the same width. You're lean and, most likely, tall. Your muscles tend to become more defined, but not much bigger, as they get stronger. Ectomorphs usually have about 16 to 22 percent body fat. Most models fall into this not-too-common category.

What's best for ectomorphs? Strength training with high resistance, few repetitions; step classes; low-impact aerobics; walking or jogging; walking up stairs; stationary biking in high gears for more resistance; and brisk walking are a few of the best body-enhancing sports for ectomorphs. Ectomorphs need to do twenty minutes of aerobic exercise three or four times a week to maintain rather than lose weight.

• **Are you an endomorph?** Curvy, sexy, you have muscles that are often hidden by body fat. Your hips are as wide as your shoulders. You are soft and womanly looking. You put on weight easily and may be a bit overweight, especially below the waist. It's hard for you to achieve a toned look because of your high body fat. Endomorphs usually have about 28 to 34 percent body fat. If your muscles bulk up from exercising, you may simply appear larger.

What's best for endomorphs? The best exercises include weight training at moderate resistance for a moderate number of repetitions;

cross-country ski machines; bicycling at a brisk pace in lower gears; power walking; running on a treadmill; and distance running. Endomorphs need to aim for forty-five to sixty minutes of aerobic exercise four to six times a week.

If you are in a state of inertia, any step, any action you can take will help alleviate the turmoil.

WAYNE DYER, *THE SKY'S THE LIMIT*

Session Thirteen "I can't do this, I don't have time, I'll start tomorrow . . . " and every other excuse you can imagine lead off this chat session. Experts say that procrastination, putting off what you know you really need to do, is a sign of fear, and Tamara tells participants that no one is more afraid of failure than an obese individual who has tried and failed before. You make up excuses because you know that starvation diets have made you feel terrible.

What kind of excuses are in your repertoire? You don't want to expend the effort or energy, and it's so much easier to say, "I don't have time to start today. I'll do it tomorrow." You may also be the greatest excuse-maker in the world because you are waiting for everything to be perfect to begin . . . aerobically exercising, eating the right foods as outlined by the perfect new diet, wearing the right exercise clothes, or whatever. "Let's face it, you may never have a perfect combination of factors," she teaches.

So, begin right now. Today. Put this book down and just do something.

When one door of happiness closes, another opens, but often we look so long at the closed door that we do not see the one that has been opened for us.

HELEN KELLER

Session Fourteen Changing your lifestyle is especially important for people with chronic health problems (heart disease, diabetes, high blood pressure, arthritis) and for the elderly, so in this session, individual cases are considered. The key idea is that even if you have a chronic health problem, you can still change your lifestyle to feel better. "No matter how old you are or what particular health condition you are dealing with, it is never too late to benefit from small positive changes in your diet and regular exercise," Tamara says. Depending on the makeup of the group, diabetes, heart disease, high blood pressure, and other topics are included here.

> *Think about your mission. Don't settle for repeating the beliefs your parents had while you were growing up. Take responsibility for developing your own ideas and conclusions.*
>
> JOHN CHAFFEE, PH.D., *THE THINKER'S WAY: 8 STEPS TO A RICHER LIFE*

Session Fifteen In session fifteen, participants fine-tune their personal approaches to wellness and discuss how they have adjusted routines, discarded bad habits, and changed attitudes and behaviors in their lives. Keep in mind: The real secret behind permanent weight loss has little to do with loss and everything to do with gain. What kind of new everyday personal lifestyle habits do you want to gain? "It's not that we need to be perfect individuals as far as our mental and physical health is concerned," Tamara stresses. "We just need to be aware of our own negative lifestyle behaviors and make positive changes so we can do our best to live healthier lives."

If you haven't already made choices from the "Right Now, Do It Today" selection of Love Self, Think Health, and Move It to Lose It menu, now might be a good time to turn to page 138.

Session Sixteen "In which area were you most successful? Did you experience more struggles in any one area? Has your energy level increased? Has your exercise level increased? Have you adopted some healthier eating habits?" These are questions that Tamara asks Fat Chat participants—and that you should pose to yourself. "Go ahead and weigh yourself if you can still find your scale," she says. In class, measurements are taken again, and other tools of evaluation are pulled back out for comparison. However, participants realize that any pounds or even inches lost are not as important as changes in habits. She may ask, "Are you eating many small meals every day, especially breakfast? What about water? Who is drinking more water each day?" No one leaves feeling any less than truly successful because they all know that "Small changes are always better than none."

Want to chat with Tamara and tell her about your progress? You can reach her at hilltk@bellsouth.net or visit her Fat Chat with Tamara website at www.fatchatwtamara.com. Or you can write to her at Fat Chat with Tamara, c/o Tamara Hill, 4014 Pinnacle Way, Hephzibah, Georgia 30815. You should definitely get in touch if you are interested in starting a Fat Chat group in your area.

Right Now, Do It Today

Move It to Lose It:

Sit up straight. Good posture burns more calories than slouching.

Walk around your neighborhood.

Regular exercise improves appetite control.

Go dancing.

Do your errands on foot.

Stop making excuses.

Put the TV remote control down.

Take the stairs instead of the elevator or escalator.

Vacuum. (Mmmmm, so good for upper-arm strength.)

Pull weeds in your yard.

Get out of the car at that drive-through restaurant.

Wash your own car.

Call a friend and meet to move.

Walk the dog.

Park in the very last row at the grocery store.

Carry in one bag at a time when you return home with your purchases.

Fidget. Even squirming in your chair helps.

Find a friendly gym.

Look for a nonthreatening aerobics instructor who will make you smile.

Look for a pretty park to explore.

Take a tennis lesson.

Explore a new sport: golf, swimming, biking.

Stand up.

Stretch.

Weight train two to three times a week.

Find an exercise that is really fun.

Look for a friend who will keep you moving.

Physical inactivity is linked to obesity.

Exercise will benefit your body anytime and anywhere.

Think Health:

Eat in front of others. It discourages bad habits.

Get your proper amount of sleep; you'll be more energetic during the day.

Don't starve. Unhealthier food choices are made when you are overly hungry.

Sometimes when you think you are hungry, you're really thirsty.

Find a good book that helps you gauge calorie content and fat grams in favorite foods.

Eat breakfast every day so you turn on your body's metabolism right away.

Go for low fat *most* of the time. (Save the high fat for special occasions.)

Unused calories are stored as fat.

The only reason to lose weight is for your health.

Learn how to read a nutrition label.

Take twenty minutes to eat a meal. (Give your body and brain time to recognize those signs of fullness.)

Eat two healthy snacks every single day.

Eat lots of fruits and vegetables. (Aim for five servings daily.)

Start drinking more water. (Build up to six to eight eight-ounce glasses a day.)

Don't deny yourself that Big Mac today. (Cut it in half and share it with someone.)

Go for all-fruit jam instead of the high-sugar kinds.

Choose sorbet, nonfat frozen yogurt, or nonfat ice cream over high-fat ice cream.

Use ground turkey in recipes calling for ground beef (meat loaf, meatballs, hamburgers).

Love Self:

Make changes you can live with.

Never deprive yourself.

Make "slow and steady" your motto. (Lose no more than two or three pounds a week.)

Be patient.

Reward yourself with a special gift rather than food.

Never look back. (Guilt is an absolute waste of time and energy.)

Enjoy this journey . . . don't endure it.

Read, read, read . . . good books and articles about health.

Pencil in time for personal fun today, not tomorrow.

Smile . . . even when you don't feel like it. The very act can change your attitude.

Stand up straight.

Stop comparing yourself to others.

Don't be obsessed with those three numbers on the scale.

Positive thoughts and feelings lead to positive results.

Sometimes less is better.

Setting unrealistic goals will probably set you up for failure.

Your goal should be "control."

Resources

These organizations will supply you with additional information about health and fitness. Call or write:

Aerobics and Fitness Association of America
15250 Ventura Boulevard, Suite 200
Sherman Oaks, CA 91403
(800) 446-2322

American College of Sports Medicine
401 W. Michigan Street
Indianapolis, IN 46202-3233
(317) 637-9200

American Council on Exercise
5820 Oberlin Drive, Suite 102
San Diego, CA 92121-3787
(800) 234-9229

American Diabetes Association
One Corporate Square, Suite 127
Atlanta, GA 30329
(404) 320-7100

American Heart Association
7320 Greenville Avenue
Dallas, TX 75231
(213) 373-6300

Aquatic Exercise Association
P.O. Box 1609
Nokomis, FL 34274-1609
(941) 486-8600

Center for Science in the Public Interest
(*Nutrition Action* newsletter)
1875 Connecticut Avenue NW, #300
Washington, DC 20009-5728
(202) 332-9110

International Association of Fitness Professionals
6190 Cornerstone Court East, Suite 204
San Diego, CA 92121
(619) 535-8979

National Dance-Exercise Instructors Training Association
1503 S. Washington Avenue, Suite 208
Minneapolis, MN 55454-1037
(612) 340-1306

National Weight Control Registry
600 Iroquois Building
3600 Forbes Avenue
Pittsburgh, PA 15213-3489
(412) 624-5353

SpeakOn (Tamara's speakers' agency)
Michael Freeman
4342 Mandalay Drive
Lilburn, GA 30047
(770) 490-5679

Stanford Arthritis Center
1000 Welch Road, Suite 204
Palo Alto, CA 94304
(415) 723-7935

ADDITIONAL READING

ACSM Fitness Book, American College of Sports Medicine (Leisure Press)

The Arthritis Helpbook, Fourth Edition (Addison Wesley)

The Complete Book of Food Counts (Dell)

Controlling Your Fat Tooth (Workman)

Dieting for Dummies (IDG Books Worldwide)

Dieting with the Duchess (Simon & Schuster)

Fat Is a Feminist Issue (Berkeley)

Fight Fat (Rodale)

Fitness for Dummies (IDG Books Worldwide)

Fitting in Fitness, American Heart Association (Times Books)

Fresh Start, The Stanford Medical School Health and Fitness Program (KQED Books)

Imagineering (McGraw-Hill)

Lose Weight with Dr. Art Ulene (Ulysses Press)

Make the Connection (Hyperion)

Overcoming Overeating (Fawcett Columbine)

The Seven Secrets of Slim People (Hay House)

Strong Women Stay Young (Bantam)

Take Care of Yourself (Addison Wesley)

Thin Is Just a Four-Letter Word (Little, Brown)

365 Ways to Get Out the Fat, American Heart Association
(Times Books)

When You Eat at the Refrigerator, Pull Up a Chair
(Hyperion)

In addition to these books, certain magazines can help you create your own individualized program. The next time you stand at a magazine rack, look for *Health, Mode, Ms. Fitness, Prevention, Sports Illustrated for Women,* or *Walking.*